Contrast-Induced Nephropathy and Nephrogenic Systemic Fibrosis

Guest Editor

SAMEH K. MORCOS, FRCS, FFRRCSI, FRCR

RADIOLOGIC CLINICS OF NORTH AMERICA

www.radiologic.theclinics.com

September 2009 • Volume 47 • Number 5

SAUNDERS an imprint of ELSEVIER, Inc.

W.B. SAUNDERS COMPANY
A Division of Elsevier Inc.

1600 John F. Kennedy Boulevard • Suite 1800 • Philadelphia, Pennsylvania 19103-2899

http://www.theclinics.com

RADIOLOGIC CLINICS OF NORTH AMERICA Volume 47, Number 5
September 2009 ISSN 0033-8389, ISBN 13: 978-1-4377-1404-3, ISBN 10: 1-4377-1404-8

Editor: Barton Dudlick

Radiologic Clinics of North America (ISSN 0033-8389) is published bimonthly by Elsevier Inc., 360 Park Avenue South, New York, NY 10010-1710. Months of issue are January, March, May, July, September, and November. Periodicals postage paid at New York, NY and additional mailing offices. Subscription prices are USD 328 per year for US individuals, USD 487 per year for US institutions, USD 160 per year for US students and residents, USD 383 per year for Canadian individuals, USD 611 per year for Canadian institutions, USD 473 per year for international individuals, USD 611 per year for international institutions, and USD 230 per year for Canadian and foreign students/residents. To receive student and resident rate, orders must be accompanied by name of affiliated institution, date of term and the signature of program/residency coordinatior on institution letterhead. Orders will be billed at individual rate until proof of status is received. Foreign air speed delivery is included in all *Clinics* subscription prices. All prices are subject to change without notice. **POSTMASTER:** Send address changes to *Radiologic Clinics of North America*, Elsevier Health Sciences Division, Subscription Customer Service, 3251 Riverport Lane, Maryland Heights, MO 63043. **Customer Service: Telephone: 1-800-654-2452** (U.S. and Canada); **1-314-447-8871** (outside U.S. and Canada). **Fax: 1-314-447-8029. E-mail: journalscustomerservice-usa@elsevier.com** (for print support); **journalsonlinesupport-usa@elsevier.com** (for online support).

Reprints. For copies of 100 or more of articles in this publication, please contact the Commercial Reprints Department, Elsevier Inc., 360 Park Avenue South, New York, New York 10010-1710. Tel.: (+1) 212-633-3812; Fax: (+1) 212-462-1935; E-mail: reprints@elsevier.com.

Radiologic Clinics of North America also published in Greek Paschalidis Medical Publications, Athens, Greece.

Radiologic Clinics of North America is covered in *MEDLINE/PubMed (Index Medicus), EMBASE/Excerpta Medica, Current Contents/Life Sciences, Current Contents/Clinical Medicine, RSNA Index to Imaging Literature, BIOSIS, Science Citation Index,* and *ISI/BIOMED.*

Printed and bound in the United Kingdom

Transferred to Digital Print 2011

Contributors

GUEST EDITOR

SAMEH K. MORCOS, FRCS, FFRRCSI, FRCR
Professor, X-ray Department, Northern General
Hospital, Sheffield, United Kingdom

AUTHORS

JERROLD L. ABRAHAM, MD
Professor of Pathology, Department of Pathology,
State University of New York, Upstate Medical
University, Syracuse, New York

JAMES G. CARIDI, MD
Associate Professor of Radiology, Department
of Radiology, University of Florida College of
Medicine, Gainesville, Florida

KYUNG J. CHO, MD, FACR
William Martel Professor of Radiology,
Department of Radiology, University of Michigan
Medical Center, Ann Arbor, Michigan

RICHARD H. COHAN, MD
Professor of Radiology, Department of Radiology,
University of Michigan Health System, Ann Arbor,
Michigan

CLAIRE COROT, PharmD, PhD
Guerbet, Research Division, Roissy, France

ANNE DENCAUSSE, PharmD, PhD
Guerbet, Research Division, Roissy, France

JAMES H. ELLIS, MD
Professor of Radiology and Urology, Department
of Radiology, University of Michigan Health
System, Ann Arbor, Michigan

IRVIN F. HAWKINS, MD
Professor of Radiology and Surgery, Department
of Radiology, University of Florida College
of Medicine, Gainesville, Florida

JEAN-MARC IDÉE, PharmD, MS
Guerbet, Research Division, Roissy, France

RICHARD W. KATZBERG, MD
Professor of Radiology, Department of Radiology,
University of California Davis Medical Center,
Sacramento, California

RAMIT LAMBA, MD
Assistant Professor of Radiology, Department
of Radiology, University of California Davis
Medical Center, Sacramento, California

ERIC LANCELOT, PharmD, PhD
Guerbet, Research Division, Roissy, France

PETER MARCKMANN, MD, DMSc
Professor, Specialist in Nephrology, Department
of Nephrology, Odense University Hospital,
Odense, Denmark

MARC PORT, PhD
Guerbet, Research Division, Roissy, France

LONE SKOV, MD, DMSc
Associate Professor, Specialist in Dermatology,
Department of Dermatology, Copenhagen
University Hospital Gentofte
Hospital, Denmark

RICHARD SOLOMON, MD, FASN
Professor, Department of Medicine, University
of Vermont School of Medicine; and
Director, Division of Hypertension and
Nephrology, Fletcher Allen Health Care,
Burlington, Vermont

CHARU THAKRAL, MD
Resident in Pathology, Department of Pathology,
State University of New York, Upstate Medical
University, Syracuse, New York

HENRIK S. THOMSEN, MD
Director and Professor of Radiology, Department
of Diagnostic Sciences, Faculty of Health Sciences,
University of Copenhagen,Copenhagen, Denmark;
and Consultant, Department of Diagnostic
Radiology, Copenhagen University Hospital
Herlev, Herlev, Denmark

Contents

> Injury to the kidney continues to occur following the administration of intravascular iodinated contrast media. In this article, the author reviews the pathophysiology of contrast-induced acute kidney injury (CIAKI), the relationship of CIAKI to long-term adverse outcomes, what type of patients are at risk of CIAKI, and how the diagnosis is made. After discussion of the reported incidence of CIAKI, an approach to prevention is briefly reviewed.

> Recent prospective clinical investigations in high-risk patients receiving intravenous contrast media for computed tomography (CT) suggest that the incidence and serious negative clinical outcomes are much less common than previously believed. Additional perspectives comparing random variations in serum creatinine in subjects not receiving contrast media show similar fluctuations that would equate to contrast-induced nephrotoxicity (CIN). Putative mechanisms for how CIN could cause death or other serious adverse clinical consequences have not been elucidated.

> Many unknowns remain concerning how best to reduce a patient's risk of contrast-induced nephropathy (CIN). Many interventions have been proposed, but few have gone unchallenged, and new questions have arisen from analysis of serum creatinine variations in patients who have not been exposed to radiographic iodinated contrast media (RICM). Use of alternate imaging tests that do not use RICM is the most direct way to avoid CIN. Hydration remains the bulwark of intervention when RICM must be administered. The administration of N-acetylcysteine is a popular pharmacologic prophylaxis against CIN but its efficacy is unclear. Hemodialysis has not been effective, but hemofiltration has shown good results in limited series.

> In the 1970s, Hawkins pioneered the intra-arterial use of carbon dioxide gas for high-risk patients who were allergic to iodinated contrast material and for those with renal failure. With the advent of digital subtraction angiography in 1980, reliable imaging of "low-density" CO_2 contrast agent became available. Subsequently, with the

addition of high-resolution of digital subtraction angiography, stacking software (adding multiple images), tilting tables and a reliable, user-friendly delivery system, CO_2 imaging has become nearly comparable to and, in some cases, superior to that of iodinated contrast media. It is the only safe contrast agent for patients in renal failure, which is extremely important in view of the increasing incidence of diabetes and complexities of interventional procedures. The low viscosity of CO_2 not only improves the sensitivities of several diagnostic procedures but may afford advantages for several interventional procedures.

Nephrogenic Systemic Fibrosis

Nephrogenic systemic fibrosis (NSF) is a new disease; the first case was diagnosed in 1997. It took 9 years before an association between NSF and gadolinium-based contrast agents (Gd-CAs) was identified. Gadolinium has several advantages for use in relation to enhanced MRI, but it is also a toxic heavy metal. For nearly 20 years, it was believed that Gd-CAs were safe, and they were used liberally. The prevalence of NSF cases varies between the various Gd-CAs, and adequate documentation of NSF cases after exposure to extracellular Gd-CAs remains a problem. All evidence points toward the fact that the real number of patients who have NSF has not been accurately totaled; the disease seems to be underdiagnosed for various reasons.

The classic hallmark symptoms of advanced nephrogenic systemic fibrosis (NSF) (skin thickening, hardening and hyperpigmentation, and disabling contractures in renal failure patients) in temporal association with Gd-based contrast agent (GBCA) exposure are almost pathognomonic of NSF. Less obvious cases may be diagnosed on the basis of history of early GBCA-related NSF symptoms (warm swellings, pain, discoloration, itching of lower legs), signs of multiorgan involvement (lungs, nervous system), the exclusion of differential diagnoses, including scleromyxedema and systemic sclerosis, and the histology of deep skin biopsies. Symptomatic treatment with intensive physiotherapy and painkillers is important, but there is no known curative medical treatment. Spontaneous remission of NSF symptoms may occur with recovery of renal function after an episode of acute renal failure, or with kidney transplantation of chronic renal failure patients.

The association between gadolinium (Gd)-containing MR imaging contrast agents and the development of nephrogenic systemic fibrosis (NSF) is well recognized. The authors review the histopathologic features, methodology, and results of analysis of tissues for Gd in NSF. Scanning electron microscopy/energy dispersive xray spectroscopy (SEM/EDS) provides sensitive detection of individual Gd-containing deposits in situ. Secondary ion mass spectroscopy has far greater sensitivity for detection of Gd than SEM/EDS and allows correlation at the cellular level. Inductively coupled plasma mass spectrometry is the recognized method for full quantitative analysis of Gd in tissues but requires destruction of the tissue and does not allow spatial correlation. In practice, the different analytic techniques provide complementary data and can be selected based on the information required.

Nephrogenic systemic fibrosis (NSF) is a highly debilitating scleroderma-like disease occurring exclusively in patients with severe or end-stage renal failure. Since the recognition of a link between gadolinium chelates (GCs) used as contrast agents for MR imaging and NSF by two independent European teams in 2006, numerous studies have described the clinical issues and investigated the mechanism of this disease. So far the most commonly reported hypothesis is based on the in vivo dechelation of GCs. The physicochemical properties of GCs, especially their thermodynamic and kinetic stabilities, are described in the present article. High kinetic stability provided by the macrocyclic structure, combined with high thermodynamic stability, minimizes the amount of free gadolinium released in the body. The current hypotheses regarding the pathophysiologic mechanism are critically discussed.

Views vary about how to avoid nephrogenic systemic fibrosis (NSF). In Europe, it is contraindicated to use gadodiamide, gadopentetate dimeglumine, and gadovertisamide in patients who have a glomerular filtration rate (GFR) of less than 30 mL/min, and these agents may only be used with caution in patients who have a GFR between 30 and 60 mL/min. Similar restrictions have not been introduced for the other six gadolinium-based contrast agents available in the European market. In the United States, the US Food and Drug Administration introduced a class ban and warned about the use of gadolinium-based contrast agents in patients who have reduced renal function. However, European and American guidelines about how to avoid NSF are generally not very different.

Radiologic Clinics of North America

THE CLINICS ARE NOW AVAILABLE ONLINE!

Access your subscription at:
www.theclinics.com

GOAL STATEMENT

The goal of the *Radiologic Clinics of North America* is to keep practicing radiologists and radiology residents up to date with current clinical practice in radiology by providing timely articles reviewing the state of the art in patient care.

ACCREDITATION

The *Radiologic Clinics of North America* is planned and implemented in accordance with the Essential Areas and Policies of the Accreditation Council for Continuing Medical Education (ACCME) through the joint sponsorship of the University of Virginia School of Medicine and Elsevier. The University of Virginia School of Medicine is accredited by the ACCME to provide continuing medical education for physicians.

The University of Virginia School of Medicine designates this educational activity for a maximum of 15 *AMA PRA Category 1 Credits*™ for each issue, 90 credits per year. Physicians should only claim credit commensurate with the extent of their participation in the activity.

The American Medical Association has determined that physicians not licensed in the US who participate in this CME activity are eligible for a maximum of *15 AMA PRA Category 1 Credits*™ for each issue, 90 credits per year.

Credit can be earned by reading the text material, taking the CME examination online at http://www.theclinics.com/home/cme, and completing the evaluation. After taking the test, you will be required to review any and all incorrect answers. Following completion of the test and evaluation, your credit will be awarded and you may print your certificate.

FACULTY DISCLOSURE/CONFLICT OF INTEREST

The University of Virginia School of Medicine, as an ACCME accredited provider, endorses and strives to comply with the Accreditation Council for Continuing Medical Education (ACCME) Standards of Commercial Support, Commonwealth of Virginia statutes, University of Virginia policies and procedures, and associated federal and private regulations and guidelines on the need for disclosure and monitoring of proprietary and financial interests that may affect the scientific integrity and balance of content delivered in continuing medical education activities under our auspices.

The University of Virginia School of Medicine requires that all CME activities accredited through this institution be developed independently and be scientifically rigorous, balanced and objective in the presentation/discussion of its content, theories and practices.

All authors/editors participating in an accredited CME activity are expected to disclose to the readers relevant financial relationships with commercial entities occurring within the past 12 months (such as grants or research support, employee, consultant, stock holder, member of speakers bureau, etc.). The University of Virginia School of Medicine will employ appropriate mechanisms to resolve potential conflicts of interest to maintain the standards of fair and balanced education to the reader. Questions about specific strategies can be directed to the Office of Continuing Medical Education, University of Virginia School of Medicine, Charlottesville, Virginia.

The faculty and staff of the University of Virginia Office of Continuing Medical Education have no financial affiliations to disclose.

The authors/editors listed below have identified no financial or professional relationships for themselves or their spouse/partner:
Kyung J. Cho, MD, FACR; Barton Dudlick (Acquisitions Editor); Richard W. Katzberg, MD; Theodore E. Keats, MD (Test Author); Ramit Lamba, MD; Peter Marckmann, MD, DMSc; Lone Skov, MD, DMSc; and Charu Thakral, MD.

The authors/editors listed below have identified the following financial or professional relationships for themselves or their spouse/partner:
Jerrold L. Abraham, MD has reviewed cases for NSF sent to him at the request of attorneys involved in litigation, and may be an expert witness in this litigation in the future.
James G. Caridi, MD is a stockholder with Angiodynamics.
Richard H. Cohan, MD has been retained by a law-firm representing GE Healthcare.
Claire Corot, PharmD, PhD is employed by Guerbet.
Anne Dencausse, PharmD, PhD is employed by Guerbet.
James H. Ellis, MD is co-investigator without salary on a funded grant with GE Healthcare, and is a consultant to legal firm representing GE Healthcare.
Irvin F. Hawkins, MD owns stock in Angiodynamics.
Jean-Marc Idée PharmD, MS is employed by Guerbet.
Eric Lancelot, PharmD, PhD is employed by Guerbet.
Sameh K. Morcos, FRCS, FFRRCSI, FRCR (Guest Editor) is on the Speakers Bureau for Bayer Schering and Bracco, and is an industry funded research/investigator and is on the Speakers Bureau for Guerbet.
Marc Port, PhD is employed by Guerbet.
Richard Solomon, MD, FASN is an industry funded research/investigator, consultant, and serves on the Speakers Bureau for Covidien and Bracco Diagnostics.
Henrik S. Thomsen, MD serves on the Advisory Board and is a patent holder with CMC Contrast AB.

Disclosure of Discussion of Non-FDA Approved Uses for Pharmaceutical Products and/or Medical Devices.
The University of Virginia School of Medicine, as an ACCME provider, requires that all faculty presenters identify and disclose any off-label uses for pharmaceutical and medical device products. The University of Virginia School of Medicine recommends that each physician fully review all the available data on new products or procedures prior to clinical use.

TO ENROLL

To enroll in the *Radiologic Clinics of North America* Continuing Medical Education program, call customer service at 1-800-654-2452 or sign up online at http://www.theclinics.com/home/cme. The CME program is available to subscribers for an additional annual fee USD 205.

Preface

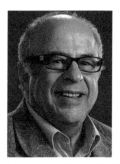

Sameh K. Morcos, FRCS, FFRRCSI, FRCR
Guest Editor

This issue of *Radiologic Clinics of North America* is dedicated to two important complications associated with the intravascular use of contrast media: contrast-induced nephropathy (CIN) and nephrogenic systemic fibrosis (NSF). The incidence, risk factors, pathophysiology, and prevention of these serious adverse effects of contrast agents are covered by renowned experts in the field of contrast media. The role of carbon dioxide as an alternative contrast agent to iodinated contrast media to avoid CIN also is addressed in this issue by a group of authors who have extensive experience in this technique.

Good understanding of the different aspects of CIN and NSF is crucial for clinicians dealing with patients suffering from renal impairment. Every effort should be made to avoid these complications in this vulnerable group of patients.

I have been fortunate in successfully recruiting a group of eminent authors for this issue of *Radiologic Clinics of North America*. Each article is written clearly and provides comprehensive coverage of the topic under consideration. The authors also provided personal views on some contentious issues based on their deep understanding of the subject and familiarity with the published literature.

I am most grateful to all the authors who made my job as editor of this issue easy and enjoyable.

Finally, I hope you will enjoy reading this issue and find the content informative and helpful for your clinical practice.

Sameh K. Morcos, FRCS, FFRRCSI, FRCR
X-ray Department
Northern General Hospital
Herries Road
Sheffield S5 7AU, UK

E-mail address:
Sameh.Morcos@sth.nhs.uk (S.K. Morcos)

Radiol Clin N Am 47 (2009) xi
doi:10.1016/j.rcl.2009.07.001

Contrast-Induced Acute Kidney Injury (CIAKI)

Richard Solomon, MD, FASN[a,b],*

KEYWORDS

- Contrast • Acute kidney injury • Creatinine
- Risk factors • Prophylaxis

Contrast media cause injury to the kidney through two complimentary mechanisms (**Fig. 1**). Contrast media cause direct injury to the cells lining the renal tubule. The injury can be reproduced in vitro by incubating cells of the proximal tubule with contrast media.[1] Cell death begins within minutes of exposure. The contrast media is taken up into the cells and alters mitochondrial function resulting in generation of reactive oxygen species and apoptosis.[2] This injury is exacerbated by a simultaneous reduction in medullary blood flow that occurs in vivo resulting from vasoconstriction of the vasa recta.[2,3] The medulla of the kidney has both very high oxygen consumption supporting active sodium transport and low tissue oxygen levels.[4] Critical tissue hypoxia results following contrast media leading to additional damage of tubule cells within this region of the kidney.

CONTRAST-INDUCED ACUTE KIDNEY INJURY IS ASSOCIATED WITH ADVERSE EVENTS

The occurrence of contrast-induced acute kidney injury (CIAKI) is associated with both short- and long-term adverse outcomes. Following cardiac angiography, in-hospital and 1-year mortality increase two- to fivefold in patients experiencing CIAKI compared with those without CIAKI.[5-7] Similar relative increases in mortality have been seen in patients with CIAKI following CT examinations, although the absolute mortality rates are far lower.[8,9] CIAKI is also predictive of the need for dialysis and long-term loss of kidney function in

some populations.[10] Recently, the association between CIAKI and long-term adverse events has been explored using data from a randomized prospective trial in which the two interventions being compared did not themselves have any potential impact on long-term adverse events. A parallel decline in CIAKI incidence and long-term adverse events in one arm of the trial supports the hypothesis that CIAKI in some way *causes* the long-term adverse events.[11]

DETERMINING WHEN CONTRAST-INDUCED ACUTE KIDNEY INJURY OCCURS

Currently, kidney injury is diagnosed when kidney function, ie, glomerular filtration rate (GFR), falls. A change in kidney function is used as a defining threshold because markers of kidney injury are not available at the current time. Such injury markers would be analogous to myocardial troponins released during myocardial injury. Creatinine is the most widely used clinical marker of GFR. An increase in serum creatinine of 25% or more or 0.5 mg/dL or more occurring within 48 to 72 hours following contrast exposure has been the traditional definition of CIAKI.[12] In an individual patient, these definitions lead to different thresholds of GFR loss required for diagnosis of CIAKI. For patients with a baseline serum creatinine lower than 2.0 mg/dL, more patients will be identified as having a kidney injury if one uses the 25% or more definition.[13] Recently, the AKIN (Acute Kidney Injury Network) has defined the first stage of

Consulting agreements – Bracco Diagnostics, Inc; Covidien.

[a] Department of Medicine, University of Vermont School of Medicine, 1 South Prospect Street, Burlington, VT 05401, USA

[b] Division of Hypertension and Nephrology, Fletcher Allen Health Care, Burlington, VT 05401, USA

* Corresponding author. Department of Medicine, University of Vermont School of Medicine, 1 South Prospect Street, Burlington, VT 05401.

E-mail address: richard.solomon@vtmednet.org

Radiol Clin N Am 47 (2009) 783–788
doi:10.1016/j.rcl.2009.06.001

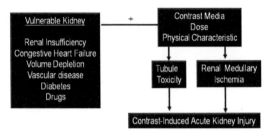

Fig. 1. Pathophysiologic mechanisms contributing to contrast-induced acute kidney injury. In the presence of a vulnerable kidney, contrast media induces sufficient direct tubule toxicity and medullary ischemia to result in a decline in glomerular filtration rate. The decline in glomerular filtration rate identifies those with acute kidney injury.

kidney injury with a rise in serum creatinine of 0.3 mg/dL or higher over 48 hours.[14] A rise in creatinine of this magnitude predicts in-hospital adverse events.[15] However, there are a number of problems with serum creatinine measurements. Serum creatinine is not only determined by glomerular filtration but also by the infusion of saline solutions, extracorporeal dialysis, and secretion by the cells lining the proximal tubule (the same cells injured by contrast media). Indeed, the variability in serum creatinine measurements in hospitalized patients may create a lot of "noise" reducing our ability to diagnose acute kidney injury when it occurs.[16] In addition, it may take 24 to 72 hours before the serum creatinine rises sufficiently to reach the threshold for diagnosis of acute kidney injury. This is because the creatinine retained when glomerular filtration is reduced must distribute in total body water, the level in serum rising relatively slowly. The rate of rise depends on the baseline level of kidney function and the severity of the injury.[17] Other markers of GFR such as cystatin C are more sensitive and specific for acute kidney injury but are not used widely in clinical practice.[18,19] Cystatin C is distributed only in extracellular volume and the serum level will rise faster than creatinine when filtration is reduced.[20] Using Cystatin C changes to define when GFR falls also results in a higher incidence of CIAKI without loss of the ability to predict long-term adverse events.[11]

Progress is being made toward identifying specific markers of kidney injury rather than function. A number of markers are currently being studied, such as NGAL, KIM-1, IL-18, but have yet to be fully validated. A clinically meaningful marker will need to reflect histologic injury to cells *and* be predictive of adverse events such as the need for dialysis or long-term loss of kidney function, mortality, rehospitalization, and so forth.

WHO IS AT RISK FOR CONTRAST-INDUCED ACUTE KIDNEY INJURY?

There is a spectrum of risk for CIAKI that reflects the mechanisms of injury induced by contrast media. Contrast media is eliminated through the kidneys. As noted above, the direct toxic effect of contrast on renal cells is exacerbated by the reduction in blood flow to the medullary portion of the kidney. Thus, patients with a decreased GFR (resulting in a greater load of contrast to be excreted by each nephron), volume depletion (reduced flow through the nephron resulting in higher concentration of contrast and longer contact time with renal cells), congestive heart failure, hypotension or volume depletion (reducing baseline renal blood flow increasing the sensitivity to contrast-induced medullary ischemia) and diabetes, use of diuretics or nonsteroidal anti-inflammatory drugs (NSAIDS) (which interfere with normal compensatory mechanisms to protect against ischemia) are at higher risk. Diabetes is associated with impaired endothelial function with loss of ability to generate nitric oxide (NO). This compromises the ability of the kidney vasculature to maintain blood flow in the face of medullary constriction induced by contrast media.[21] In addition to these patient-specific risk factors, procedure-specific factors include the amount of contrast administered grams of iodine/estimated glomerular filtration rate and the route of administration (intravenous versus intra-arterial).

WHAT IS THE INCIDENCE OF CONTRAST-INDUCED ACUTE KIDNEY INJURY?

There is support for a higher incidence of CIAKI (using current serum creatinine definitions) with intra-arterial compared with intravenous contrast administration. Possible reasons for this higher incidence of CIAKI include a greater dose of contrast administered with coronary interventions (from which most of the intra-arterial data are derived), a greater burden of underlying cardiovascular disease in patients who receive intra-arterial contrast, a greater likelihood of hemodynamic compromise at the time of intra-arterial injection in patients (particularly those with urgent cardiac catheterizations), and finally the likelihood of atheromatous emboli in patients receiving intra-arterial contrast.

For intra-arterial contrast administration, a risk-profiling score has been developed and validated by Mehran and colleagues.[22] This scoring system gives points for the amount of contrast administered, the baseline level of GFR, hemodynamic instability, congestive heart failure, age of patient, and presence of anemia and diabetes. Four categories of risk are defined based on the sum of the points. The incidence of CIAKI increases from 8% to 57% as the risk category increases. In this model, the risk increases as GFR falls below 60 mL/min/1.73 m^2.

For intravenous (IV) contrast administration specifically, the primary risk factors are eGFR, dose of contrast, and setting (inpatient versus outpatient).[9] The risk of CIAKI in outpatients increases significantly when eGFR is less than 45 mL/min.[1]

HOW DOES KNOWLEDGE OF THE PATHOGENESIS OF CONTRAST-INDUCED ACUTE KIDNEY INJURY LEAD TO EFFECTIVE PREVENTION THERAPIES?

Prevention of CIAKI means (1) reducing the kidney injury and (2) the adverse outcomes associated with such an injury. To date, there are no data regarding reducing injury and relatively little data addressing long-term adverse outcomes. All the "evidence" regarding prevention of CIAKI is derived from trials looking at changes in serum creatinine, an imperfect marker of CIAKI. These trials can be categorized into studies of (1) intravenous volume supplementation (frequently referred to as "hydration"), (2) pharmacologic agents to increase renal blood flow, (3) pharmacologic agents to reduce the generation of reactive oxygen species, and (4) extracorporeal strategies to remove contrast from the body and (5) differences between contrast agents in the incidence of CIAKI. The vast majority of prospective randomized clinical trials have been conducted in patients undergoing cardiac angiography; relatively few trials have included patients receiving intravenous contrast. These trials have infrequently reported follow-up data on adverse effects. The details of the different strategies to reduce the risk of CIAKI are discussed elsewhere in this issue. Only a concise overview is presented in this article with some emphasis on how to reduce the risk of CIAKI after intravenous administration of contrast media.

- Intravenous volume expansion is considered the standard strategy for prevention of CIAKI in high-risk patients exposed to contrast. Although there are no randomized controlled trials (RCTs) of such strategy specifically with intravenous contrast, there is an indication of the role of "hydration" from clinical trials of contrast media comparisons in patients undergoing MDCT. Three recent trials in high-risk patients with an average eGFR of 45 mL/min found an incidence of CIAKI of 5% (defined as a ≥25% increase in serum creatinine at 48 hours post contrast) despite the minimal use of any intravenous fluids before, during, or after contrast exposure. These data are consistent with the observational data of Weisbord and colleagues[9] suggesting that less than 7% and 50% of patients with eGFR lower than 60 mL/min undergoing CT examinations in the outpatient and inpatient setting respectively received any intravenous fluid.

- All attempts to reduce the incidence of CIAKI with systemic administration of vasodilators have failed in multicenter clinical trials. No trials have involved intravenous contrast administration. Reasons for such failure include the often hypotensive effects of these agents resulting in exacerbation of the medullary vasoconstriction produced by the contrast medium and the use of vasoconstrictive antagonists that lacked specificity for the renal receptors within the medullary portion of the kidney.

- The original publication showing efficacy of antioxidant therapy (N-acetylcysteine) for prevention of CIAKI involved patients with severe renal dysfunction (eGFR <30 mL/min) undergoing abdominal CT with 75 mL of low-osmolality contrast media.[23] Subsequent single-center trials involved patients undergoing coronary angiography with larger doses of contrast media. Multiple meta-analyses have suggested that N-acetycysteine is not effective, at least in the same doses as used in the seminal trial.[24] However, higher doses of N-acetylcysteine appear to have greater efficacy. N-acetycysteine is also effective in vitro in preventing cell apoptosis.[1,25,26] Thus, although based on only one small single-center trial, N-acetylcysteine should be considered a potentially effective prophylaxis in high-risk patients undergoing CT examination.

- Infusion of sodium bicarbonate is another antioxidant strategy frequently used in patients with baseline renal insufficiency undergoing cardiac angiography. The generation of reactive oxygen species is facilitated in an acid environment as might occur in the distal nephron. Administration of sodium bicarbonate or acetazolamide will alkalinize the urine and presumably slow down the generation of these toxic oxygen species. Multiple single-center trials in these patients have also produced conflicting results but recent meta-analyses suggest a benefit[27] particularly in patients

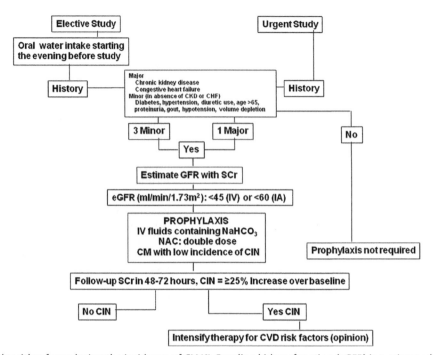

Fig. 2. An algorithm for reducing the incidence of CIAKI. Baseline kidney function (eGFR) is a primary determinant of the risk of CIAKI and differs between those receiving intravenous versus intra-arterial contrast. The difference may be related to the dose of contrast administered, ie, the ratio of contrast given (gI) to eGFR. Because more contrast is generally given with intra-arterial administration, the threshold for increasing risk for CIAKI starts at a higher level of eGFR. Bicarbonate and N-acetylcysteine therapy is recommended for the high-risk patients, not because of compelling evidence of efficacy from clinical trials but because of their safety, low cost, and ease of administration. New definitions of CIAKI are currently being explored. Cystatin C may replace serum creatinine in the near future.

undergoing emergency studies.[28] However, despite a reduction in the incidence of CIAKI, there was no effect on hard outcomes, such as need for renal replacement therapy or mortality.[28] None of these trials have involved patients exposed to *intravenous* contrast media. Because N-acetylcysteine and sodium bicarbonate may act in different ways to reduce oxidative injury, their combination might be more efficacious than either used alone. Support for this approach has been reported in patients undergoing cardiac angiography.[29] Other studies, including meta-analyses, found no benefit to the combination of N-acetylcysteine and bicarbonate.[30]

- Hemodialysis and hemofiltration have been studied in high-risk patients undergoing cardiac angiography.[31] For the most part, these therapies are ineffective, labor intensive, and costly. This approach needs validation in a larger group of patients and by other investigators before adoption by the larger medical community.

- Differences between contrast agents could exist and be related to the different physical properties of the agents—osmolality, viscosity, iconicity, and molecular size.
- However, there are no conclusive data to support differences in the incidence of CIAKI between a number of low-osmolality contrast media and iso-osmolality contrast media.[32–35]

SUMMARY

Injury to renal cells occurs during exposure to contrast media. Our ability to detect such injury clinically is limited. The use of an imperfect marker of kidney function (serum creatinine) may result in a false sense of safety, as only the "tip of the iceberg" is being exposed by such measurements. Until further data are available, it is reasonable to screen for high-risk patients using (1) eGFR, (2) hospital versus outpatient setting (for IV contrast administration), (3) presence of hemodynamic instability, and (4) dose of contrast to be administered. A strategy for prevention in these high-risk patients is outlined in **Fig. 2.**

REFERENCES

1. Romano G, Briguori C, Quintavalle C, et al. Contrast agents and renal cell apoptosis. Eur Heart J 2008; 29:2569–76.
2. Persson BP, Hansell P, Liss P. Pathophysiology of contrast medium-induced nephropathy. Kidney Int 2005;68:14–22.
3. Sendeski M, Patzak A, Pallone TL, et al. Iodixanol, constriction of medullary descending vasa recta, and risk for contrast medium-induced nephropathy. Radiology 2009;251:697–704.
4. Heyman SN, Brezis M, Reubinoff CA, et al. Acute renal failure with selective medullary injury in the rat. J Clin Invest 1988;82:401–12.
5. Gruberg L, Mintz GS, Mehran R, et al. The prognostic implications of further renal function deterioration within 48 h of interventional coronary procedures in patients with pre-existent chronic renal insufficiency. J Am Coll Cardiol 2000;36: 1542–8.
6. McCullough PA, Wolyn R, Rocher LL, et al. Acute renal failure after coronary intervention: incidence, risk factors, and relationship to mortality. Am J Med 1997;103:368–75.
7. Rihal CS, Textor SC, Grill DE, et al. Incidence and prognostic importance of acute renal failure after percutaneous coronary intervention. Circulation 2002;105:2259–64.
8. Levy EM, Viscoli CM, Horwitz RI. The effect of acute renal failure on mortality. A cohort analysis. JAMA 1996;275:1489–94.
9. Weisbord S, Mor MK, Resnick AL, et al. Incidence and outcomes of contrast-induced AKI following computed tomography. Clin J Am Soc Nephrol 2008;3:1274–81.
10. Ijak F, Yousaf M, Sohail I, et al. Long term renal consequences of acute kidney injury related to contrast media. J Am Soc Nephrol 2006;17:280A.
11. Solomon R, Mehran R, Natarajan MK, et al. Contrast-induced nephropathy and long-term adverse events: cause and effect? Clin J Am Soc Nephrol 2009;4:1162–9.
12. Solomon R, Barrett B. Follow-up of patients with contrast-induced nephropathy. Kidney Int 2006;69: S46–50.
13. Solomon R, Segal AS. Defining acute kidney injury: what is the most appropriate metric? Nature Clin Pract Nephrol 2008;4:208–15.
14. Mehta RL, Kellum JA, Shah SV, et al. Acute kidney injury network (AKIN): report of an initiative to improve outcomes in acute kidney injury. Crit Care 2007;11:R31.
15. Chertow GM, Soroko SH, Paganini EP, et al. Mortality after acute renal failure: models for prognostic stratification and risk adjustment. Kidney Int 2006;70: 1120–6.
16. Newhouse J, Kho D, Rao QA, et al. Frequency of serum creatinine changes in the absence of iodinated contrast material: implications for studies of contrast nephrotoxicity. Am J Radiol 2008;191: 376–82.
17. Waikar SS, Bonventre JV. Creatinine kinetics and the definition of acute kidney injury. J Am Soc Nephrol 2009;20:672–9.
18. Herget-Rosenthal S, Marggraf G, Husing J, et al. Early detection of acute renal failure by serum cystatin C. Kidney Int 2004;66:1115–22.
19. Kato K, Sato N, Yamamoto T, et al. Valuable markers for contrast-induced nephropathy in patients undergoing cardiac catheterization. Circ J 2008;72: 1499–505.
20. Herget-Rosenthal S, Pietruck F, Volbracht L, et al. Serum cystatin C: a superior marker of rapidly reduced glomerular filtration after uninephrectomy in kidney donors compared to creatinine. Clin Nephrol 2005;64:41–6.
21. Economides PA, Caselli A, Zuo CS, et al. Kidney oxygenation during water diuresis and endothelial function in patients with type 2 diabetes and subjects at risk to develop diabetes. Metabolism 2004;53:222–7.
22. Mehran R, Aymong ED, Nikolsky E, et al. A simple risk score for prediction of contrast-induced nephropathy after percutaneous coronary intervention: development and initial validation. J Am Coll Cardiol 2004;44:1393–9.
23. Tepel M, Van Der Giet M, Schwarzfeld C, et al. Prevention of radiographic-contrast-agent-induced reductions in renal function by acetylcysteine. N Engl J Med 2000;343:180–4.
24. Gonzales D, Norsworthy KJ, Kern SJ, et al. A meta-analysis of N-acetylcysteine in contrast-induced nephrotoxicity: unsupervised clustering to resolve heterogeneity. BMC Med 2007;5:32–45.
25. Briguori C, Columbo A, Violante A, et al. Standard vs double dose of N-acetylcysteine to prevent contrast agent associated nephrotoxicity. Eur Heart J 2004; 25:206–11.
26. Marenzi G, Assanelli E, Marana I, et al. N-Acetylcysteine and contrast-induced nephropathy in primary angioplasty. N Engl J Med 2006;354:2773–82.
27. Joannidis M, Schmid M, Wiedermann CJ. Prevention of contrast media-induced nephropathy by isotonic sodium bicarbonate: a meta-analysis. Wien Klin Wochenschr 2008;120:742–8.
28. Meier P, Ko DT, Tamura A, et al. Sodium bicarbonate-based hydration prevents contrast-induced nephropathy: a meta-analysis. BMC Med 2009;7:23–34.

29. Briguori C, Airoldi F, D'Andrea D, et al. Renal insufficiency following contrast media administration trial (REMEDIAL). A randomized comparison of 3 preventive strategies. Circulation 2007;115:1211–7.

30. Navaneethan S, Singh S, Appasamy S, et al. Sodium bicarbonate therapy for prevention of contrast-induced nephropathy: a systematic review and meta-analysis. Am J Kidney Dis 2008;53:617–27.

31. Deray G. Dialysis and iodinated contrast media. Kidney Int 2006;69:S25–9.

32. Barrett B, Thomsen H, Katzberg R. Nephrotoxicity of low-osmolar iopamidol vs iso-osmolar iodixanol in renally impaired patients: the IMPACT study. Invest Radiol 2006;41:815–21.

33. Kuhn M, Chen N, Sahani DV, et al. The PREDICT study: a randomized double-blind comparison of contrast-induced nephropathy after low- or isoosmolar contrast agent exposure. Am J Radiol 2008;191: 151–7.

34. Nguyen S, Suranyi P, Ravenel JG, et al. Iso-osmolality versus low-osmolality iodinated contrast medium at intravenous contrast-enhanced CT: effect on kidney function. Radiology 2008;248: 97–105.

35. Thomsen HS, Morcos SK, Erley CM, et al. Investigators in the Abdominal Computed Tomography: IO-MERON 400 Versus VISIPAQUE 320 Enhancement (ACTIVE) Study. The ACTIVE Trial: comparison of the effects on renal function of iomeprol-400 and iodixanol-320 in patients with chronic kidney disease undergoing abdominal computed tomography. Invest Radiol 2008;43:170–8.

Contrast-Induced Nephropathy after Intravenous Administration: Fact or Fiction?

Richard W. Katzberg, MD*, Ramit Lamba, MD

KEYWORDS

- Contrast media • Kidney injury • Kidney function
- CT • Acute renal failure

It has been over a half century since the first episode of contrast-induced nephrotoxicity (CIN) was reported by Bartels and colleagues,[1] a case report occurring following intravenous pyelography with 20 mL of Diodrast 50% in a 69-year-old male with marked albuminuria, unknown baseline renal function, multiple myeloma and treatment with fluid restriction. Since then, there have been several thousand clinical reports, the rate of which accelerated appreciably in the mid-1970s, in part in parallel with increases in both intra-arterial and intravenous use.[2]

The major driving forces in the development of contrast media (CM) have been to eliminate systemic and central nervous system toxicities rather than renal toxicity.[3–7] Indeed, with the advent of nonionic, low-osmolality contrast media (LOCM) in the 1980s, most general adverse events have been significantly reduced and require no medical treatment.[8] For example, severe or life-threatening reactions to nonionic monomeric CM occur in association with approximately 4 in 10,000 examinations and with a mortality rate estimated to be approximately 1 in 170,000 examinations, a remarkable safety profile.[8,9]

Contrast material-induced nephropathy is the sudden rapid deterioration of renal function resulting from parenteral contrast media administration *and with no alternative clinical explanation*. The incidence of CIN has been reported to range from less than 1% to greater than 30%. This wide variation in incidence is attributed to factors that include a lack of consensus in definitions, assessments based on SCr levels rather than more direct measures of kidney function, differing patient populations such as inpatients versus outpatients, wide variability in CM doses, variation in the completeness of timing of patient follow-up, and a likely variation in the patient's hydration state. In addition, there has been a paucity of comparison of the nephrotoxicity caused by CM administered by different routes (eg, intra-arterial versus intravenous). CIN is not common in patients with normal preexisting renal function; rather, it is more frequent in patients with renal impairment, especially when the renal insufficiency (RI) is attributable to diabetic nephropathy. Eighty percent to 90% of the use is with intravenous (IV), predominantly contrast-enhanced computerized tomography (CECT) and 10% to 20% for cardiac and noncardiac angiography and interventional.[10]

In this article, we assess evidence from experimental observations, clinical trials, and literature review to gain perspectives on the relative risk of CIN, expected clinical outcomes, and possible protective strategies for IV use. The major focus will be on patients who are most vulnerable, with or without diabetes.

OVERVIEW OF EXPERIMENTAL OBSERVATIONS

The pharmacokinetics of all the currently used iodinated CM are similar.[3–6] All of these agents

Department of Radiology, University of California Davis Medical Center, 4860 Y Street, Suite 3100, Sacramento, CA 95819, USA
* Corresponding author.
E-mail address: richard.katzberg@ucdmc.ucdavis.edu (R. Katzberg).

Radiol Clin N Am 47 (2009) 789–800
doi:10.1016/j.rcl.2009.06.002

have very low lipid solubility, extremely low chemical activity with bodily fluids, relatively small molecular weights, a half-time in patients with normal renal function of approximately 1 to 2 hours, and are in a class of compounds termed "extracellular tracers."

The general characteristics of iodinated CM that have significant biologic implications include osmolality, ionicity, hydrophilicity, viscosity, and the unique chemical structure.[3,6] The systemic effect of CM, predominately because of their increased osmolality, is to increase the plasma volume, decrease the hematocrit, decrease peripheral vascular resistance, increase blood flow, and decrease systemic blood pressure. There is a transient decrease in the glomerular filtration rate (GFR) as a result of osmotic effects, a physiologic response seen with all nonspecific osmotic diuretics such as mannitol.[6,11]

Contrast media are freely filtered without hindrance.[12] The concentration of CM in the initial filtrate is effectively the same as that in plasma, as protein binding of modern urographic contrast media is negligible. Because molecules of CM, like those of mannitol, are not reabsorbed, they continue to exert an osmotic force, reducing the reabsorption of water from the tubules. The contrast-induced inductions in GFR, filtration fraction, and renal perfusion are explainable on the bases of intratubular and intracapsular pressure changes cause by the hypertonic solution. On the basis of Starling's law, the increase in proximal tubular hydrostatic pressure decreases the gradient for filtration from the glomerular capillary. These effects are markedly attenuated when the LOCM and iso-osmolar contrast media (IOCM) are used.

As a potential etiologic factor in CIN, the greatest amount of recent clinical attention has focused on the hemodynamic effects of CM. Interest in the hemodynamic pathway was stimulated by prior animal investigations that included an assessment of effects of high osmolar contrast media (HOCM) on renal blood flow with an initial increase followed by a decrease. This observation initiated the hypothesis that ischemia is the likely candidate for the cause of CIN. However, the predominate hemodynamic response with the *intravenous bolus injection of CM* is only a vasodilatation. This finding has been documented in both animal and human studies.[13] Weisberg and colleagues[14] observed an increase in renal blood flow in humans. In addition, Guevera and colleagues[15] also showed an increase in renal blood flow following the intravenous administration of contrast agents in patients with cirrhosis of the liver.

On the other hand, an additional hypothesis on the hemodynamic effects of contrast media is that there is a masked decrease in blood flow in the medullary thick ascending limb of the nephron and consequent acute renal injury. However, Agmon and colleagues[16] and Lancelot and colleagues[17] demonstrated an increase in medullary renal blood flow after CM administration in rats. The one exception was a demonstration of a decrease in medullary blood flow with the IOCM.

There have been multiple attempts to develop animal models that simulate the clinical findings for CIN. However, none of these have been successful using doses of contrast media that are within clinical ranges. The most methodical attempt to develop CIN was by Vaamonde and colleagues[18] In this rigorous study, both the acute and chronic renal effects of the intravenous injection of an ionic HOCM were (osmolality 1650 mOsm/kg) studied in diabetic and age-matched normal rats. Four protocols to assess risk factors in both the diabetic and control rats were used: adult rats with normal hydration; old dehydrated rats with diabetes mellitus of long duration; rats with prior decreased creatinine clearance (remnant kidney); and diabetic rats treated with insulin. The anticipated decrease in GFR was noted within 20 minutes after the intravenous injection of meglumine diatrizoate sodium 76% and with stabilization to baseline levels in both the control and diabetic animals. The authors concluded that the diabetic state alone, or in combination with hydropenia and old age do not appear to confer an enhanced sensitivity to the renal effects of IV contrast medium administration.

ADMINISTRATION OF NONIONIC LOW- AND ISO-OSMOLAR CONTRAST: NEW PROSPECTIVE STUDIES WITH INTRAVENOUS CONTRAST MEDIA FOR COMPUTERIZED TOMOGRAPHY

Recent prospective studies employing the use of IV contrast media in patients with RI and diabetes mellitus have provided new insights into the relative rate of CIN in those patients being evaluated with CECT. The great majority of previous reports on CIN have been forthcoming from clinical observations in the cardiac catheterization laboratory. Tables 1–2 show a list of the recent prospective studies for CECT and show an overall incidence of CIN with the current generation of LOCM to be at the *5.1% rate*. These results allow apples-to-apples IV comparisons and now with a reasonably large database. The studies by Tepel and colleagues,[19] Nguyen and colleagues,[20] and Weisbord and colleagues[21] are single center investigations. The studies by Barrett and

Table 1
Contrast-induced nephrotoxicity and intravenous contrast media in renal insufficient patients

Study	Agents	Prospective Design	Def CIN	Rates (%)
Tepel et al (2000)	LOCM	Yes	↑SCr ≥0.5 mg/dL	9/42 (21%)
Barrett et al (IMPACT, 2006)	LOCM	Yes	↑SCr ≥0.5 mg/dL	2/153 (1.3%)
Thomsen, et al (ACTIVE, 2007)	LOCM	Yes	↑SCr ≥0.5 mg/dL	5/148 (3.4%)
Kuhn et al[a] (PREDICT, 2008)	LOCM	Yes	SCr ≥25%	13/248 (5.2%)
Nguyen et al (2008)	LOCM	Yes	↑SCr ≥0.5 mg/dL	13/117 (11.1%)
Weisbord et al (2008)	LOCM	Yes	↑SCr ≥0.5 mg/dL	13/367 (3.5%)
				Subtotal 55/1075 (5.1%)

Summary
- CIN LOCM with RI 5.1%
- Controls with RI 5.9%[35]

Abbreviations: CIN, contrast-inhanced nephrotoxicity; LOCM, low-osmolality contrast media; RI, renal insufficiency; SCr, serum creatinine.
[a] All with renal insufficiency and diabetes.

colleagues,[22] Thomsen and colleagues,[23] and Kuhn and colleagues[24] are multicenter studies.[19–24] All of these studies are prospective and the criteria for CIN are uniform. All subjects have RI and there was much closer attention to acquisition of study patients with baseline stable renal function. There is a broad patient base from North America, Europe, and China. Both LOCM and IOCM were assessed. Patients with concomitant diabetes ranged from 20.2% to 100.0%.

Tepel and colleagues[19] performed a single-center prospective study involving 83 patients with chronic renal insufficiency (mean SCr level, 2.4 mg/dL ± 1.3 [SD]) who underwent CT with iopromide, a LOCM. Patients were randomly assigned to receive intravenously N-acetylcysteine NAC (600 mg orally twice) with 0.45% saline before and after CM administration or to receive placebo with saline. Our interest in this report is in the subjects who did not receive NAC. Nine (21%) of these 42 subjects had a 0.5 mg/dL increase in SCr 48 hours after CM administration. Fourteen (33%) had diabetes mellitus. The authors stated that repeated measurements during the week before CM administration revealed "only minor" changes in SCr level (mean variation, 0.1 mg/dL ± 0.3 [9 μmol/L ± 26]; $P = .12$).

Barrett and colleagues[22] in the IMPACT study compared the effects of a nonionic monomer, iopamidol-370, to a nonionic dimer, iodixanol-320,

Table 2
Serious adverse outcomes for CT contrast procedures

Study	Dialysis	Death
Tepel et al (2000)	0/42	0/42
Barrett et al (IMPACT, 2006)	0/153	0/153
Thompsen et al (ACTIVE, 2007)	0/148	0/148
Kuhn et al (PREDICT, 2008)	0/248	0/248
Nguyen et al (2008)	0/117	0/117
Weisbord et al (2008)	0/367	0/367
TOTALS	0/1075	0/1075

All prospective and renal insufficiency ± diabetes.

on renal function in patients with renal impairment who underwent contrast-enhanced multidetector CT (CE-MDCT) in a multicenter (15 centers in North America and China), double-blind, randomized, parallel group study. One hundred fifty-three patients with stable, moderate or severe chronic renal disease (SCr level $\geq$1.5 mg/dL and/or creatinine clearance 10–59 mL/min) were enrolled, and CIN was defined as an absolute increase in SCr of 0.5 mg/dL or higher. The two study groups were comparable with regard to all baseline characteristics. An absolute increase in SCr to 0.5 mg/dL or greater was observed in 2 (3%) of 76 patients who received iodixanol-320 and in none (0%) of the 7 patients who received iopamidol-370 (95% confidence interval: −6.2%, 1.0%; P = .2). The authors concluded that the rate of CIN was low and not significantly different with patients from moderate to severe kidney disease who received a nonionic monomer and those who received a nonionic dimer. Overall, 23.5% of subjects with renal insufficiency also had diabetes mellitus.

Thomsen and colleagues[23] in the ACTIVE trial compared the effects of a nonionic monomer, iomeprol-400 to a nonionic dimer, iodixanol-320 on renal function in patients with impairment who underwent CE-MDCT in another multicenter (16 centers in Europe and China), double-blind, randomized, parallel group study. One hundred and forty-eight patients with stable moderate-to-severe chronic kidney disease (SCr $\geq$1.5 mg/dL and/or calculated creatinine clearance <60 mL/mn) were randomized to equi-iodine doses (40 gl). Contrast-induced nephropathy was defined as an absolute SCr increase of 0.5 mg/dL or greater from baseline to 48 to 72 hours post dose. Mean SCr changes from baseline were also assessed. The two study groups were comparable with regard to age, gender distribution, concomitant nephrotoxins, hydration status, and total iodine dose; however, the iomeprol-400 showed a significantly higher proportion of patients with diabetes mellitus (P = .02). Five of 72 patients receiving iodixanol-320 (6.9%) and none of the patients receiving iomeprol-400 showed an increase of 0.5 mg/dL or greater from baseline (P = .025, 95% CI −12.8%, −1.1%). The mean SCr change from baseline was significantly higher (P = .017) after iodixanol-320 than after iomeprol-400. These authors concluded that the incidence of CIN was significantly higher after IV administration of iodixanol-320 than iomeprol-400. The overall rate of CIN in all study groups was 5/148 (3.4%) of patients. Overall, 30/148 (20.2%) had diabetes.

Kuhn and colleagues[24] in the PREDICT study compared the effects of a nonionic monomer iopamidol-370 to a nonionic dimer, iodixanol-320, on

renal function in patients with both renal impairment and diabetes mellitus who underwent CE-MDCT in a multicenter (23 centers in North America and China) double-blind, randomized, parallel group study. Two hundred and forty-eight patients with moderate-to-severe chronic kidney disease (estimated glomerular filtration rate [eGFR] = 20–59 mL/min/1.73 m^2) and diabetes mellitus. Again, CIN was defined as an increase in the serum creatinine level after contrast administration of 25% or greater from baseline level. The overall CIN rate was 13/248 (5.2%). Increases in serum creatinine levels of 25% or greater occurred in 7 patients (5.6%) receiving iopamidol-370 and in 6 patients (4.9%) receiving iodixanol-320 (95% CIN, −4.8% to 6.3%; P = 1.0). Also notable was that in patients with a baseline serum creatinine value of 2.0 mg/dL or higher, baseline estimated GFR of 40 mL/min/1.73 m^2 or less, or those receiving 140 mL or more of contrast medium, the incidence of CIN was low and comparable between the two contrast agents (P = 1.0 in all instances). Overall, in those patients with baseline serum creatinine value of 2.0 mg/dL or greater, no cases of CIN occurred and in those patients with a baseline estimated GFR of 40 mL/min/1.73 m^2 or less, only one case of CIN was observed.

Nguyen and colleagues[20] performed a single-center, randomized, double-blind prospective study involving 117 patients with decreased renal function and who underwent CE-MDCT with either the nonionic monomer iopromide-370 or the nonionic dimer iodixanol-320. Outcome measures were of SCr increase or GFR decrease for 3 days after CT, a SCr increase $\geq$0.5 mg/dL, a GFR reduction of 5 mL/min or greater and patient outcomes at 30 and 90 days at follow-up. Fewer patients in the iodixanol group (8.5%) than in the iopromide group (27.8%) had SCr increases of 0.5 mg/dL or higher ($\geq$25%, P = .012). Two patients in each group had SCr increases of 1.0 mg/dL or more (not significant). No patient had a contrast material-related adverse event at 30- or 90-day follow-up. Combining study groups, the overall rate of CIN was 13/117 (11.1%). Diabetes mellitus was present in 33/117 (26.5%).

Weisbord and colleagues[21] performed a single-center prospective study in patients with estimated glomerular filtration rates less than 60 mL/min per 1.73 m^2 undergoing nonemergent CE-MDCT with intravenous CM at an academic VA Medical Center. Serum creatinine was assessed 48 to 96 hours postprocedure to quantify the incidence of CIN, in a total of 421 patients. Overall, 6.5% of patients developed an increase in serum creatinine of 25% or more, and 3.5% demonstrated a rise in serum creatinine of 0.5 mg/dL or more. Although only 6% of outpatients received pre-procedure and post-procedure intravenous fluid, fewer than 1% of outpatients with estimated GFRs greater than 45 mL/min per 1.73 m^2 manifested an increase in serum creatinine greater than or equal to 0.5 mg/dL. The authors concluded that their results suggest that biochemical evidence of contrast-induced acute kidney injury (CIAKI) in clinically stable patients is not synonymous with clinically significant renal failure. They also concluded that although biochemically defined CIAKI was not uncommon in their study population, serious adverse outcomes were rare. None of their patients required dialysis, and there were no associations with CIAKI with need for hospital admission or death at 30 days. Forty-one percent of their patients had both renal insufficiency and diabetes mellitus. The overall incidence of CIN was 13/367 (3.5%).

These investigators also assessed the incidence of CIAKI based on the RIFLE criteria, which defines acute kidney injury (AKI) based on 5 distinct categories: Risk, Injury, Failure, Loss, and End-stage kidney disease. RIFLE criteria were developed to standardize the diagnosis of acute renal failure and the term AKI was proposed to encompass the entire spectrum from minor changes in renal function to requirement for renal replacement therapy.[25,26]

Using RIFLE criteria, an insult would be considered renal injury if there were a biochemical evidence of an increase in serum creatinine by a factor of 2 (100%). Most definitions of CIN, however, use a serum creatinine increase of 1.25 (25%), which would result in categorizing more patients as having CIN, in contrast to the higher thresholds for injury based on the RIFLE criteria. In the Weisbord and colleagues[21] study, only 2 patients (0.5%) met criteria for Risk stage of AKI (increase in SCr times 1.5) using the RIFLE definition. None of their patients met criteria for more advanced stages. The authors recommended that future study designs for CT and CIN should enroll larger numbers of high-risk subjects and incorporate outcomes such as need for dialysis and/or death in sample size estimates.

In summary, the combined overall rate of CIN in patients with renal insufficiency is low at approximately 5%. CIN with LOCM with renal insufficiency is 5.1% and CIN with IOCM and renal insufficiency is 4.8%. In head-to-head trials, there appears to be no significant difference between the nonionic LOCM and the nonionic IOCM.[20,22–24] Diabetes mellitus did not appear to be an independent risk factor for CIN. No single prophylactic measure could be consistently identified in any of these clinical trials, even including variable degrees of patient hydration.

CONTRAST-INDUCED NEPHROTOXICITY WITH INTRA-ARTERIAL VERSUS INTRAVENOUS ADMINISTRATION OF CONTRAST MEDIA
Contrast-induced Nephrotoxicity Rates and Adverse Clinical Outcomes

The incidence of CIN with the IV use of contrast material has been overrated for several reasons: (1) extrapolation between the cardiology experience with percutaneous catheterization and coronary intervention with contrast-enhanced multidetector CT; (2) uncertainties about cause and effect relationships; and (3) failure to take into consideration random variations in SCr fluctuations that may occur either naturally or in response to other insults.

It is interesting that a significant increase in the reported incidences of CIN, as reported by Mudge[2] was recognized by numerous reports primarily in the cardiology literature. It is surprising since in that era, HOCM were still the primary agents used, and there were little or no reports of CIN occurring with IV use. On the other hand, the mid-1970s was also a period of time in which cardiac catheterization became more prevalent. The beginning widespread use of LOCM occurred in the early to mid-1980s and multiple clinical trials with their use intravenously showed little evidence for CIN, death, or dialysis.[27]

As noted, above, the more recent prospective investigations beginning with Tepel and colleagues[19] have shown low rates of CIN, overall being approximately 5.1%.[19–24] On the other hand, the cardiology literature reports overall rates of CIN in patients with chronic kidney disease and diabetes to be in the range of one third of patients as noted by Rudnick and colleagues[28] in the large Iohexol Cooperative Study, a large randomized trial. A comparison to the latter study is the new, prospective study by Kuhn and colleagues[24] in 2008, the incidence of CIN with LOCM in patients with renal insufficiency and diabetes mellitus was 5.2% (13/248).

The rates of serious adverse outcomes between the cardiac cath experience and the CE-MDCT is even more striking. For example, Gruberg and colleagues[29] in a retrospective observational study in 439 patients with RI showed a 37.7% rate of CIN, a 7.0% rate of patients regarding dialysis, a nearly threefold (13.9% versus 4.9%) increase in in-hospital mortality, and a 22.6% mortality rate in those patients requiring dialysis.[30] This is contradistinction to the studies for CE-MDCT in RI patients of Tepel and colleagues,[19] Barrett and colleagues,[22] Thomsen and colleagues,[23] Kuhn and colleagues,[24] Nguyen and colleagues,[20] and Weisbord and colleagues[21] (see **Table 2**) where

CIN rates were 0% (0/1,075) for dialysis and with associated death rates of 0% (0/1075).

One widely quoted study that markedly deviates in the reported rates of morbidity and mortality with the intravenous use of contrast material was that by Levy and colleagues.[31] This study retrospectively analyzed the mortality findings in 16,248 inpatients who underwent contrast procedures (half of the patients underwent angiography; the other patients underwent computed tomography, and other miscellaneous contrast procedures) between 1987 and 1989 at a large academic hospital using a matched pairs cohort design. A total of 174 patients developed CIN and indexed subjects with acute kidney injury were matched with control subjects not having acute kidney injury for age, baseline, SCr, and type of contrast-enhanced procedures. The mean SCr was 1.6/mg/dL in both index and control subjects. However, when compared with control subjects, index subjects had significantly more acute comorbid conditions and the in-hospital mortality rate for an index patient was 34% compared with 7% for the matched subjects ($P \leq .001$). As noted by Rudnick and Feldman,[30] the clinical course of CIN was atypical with 29% having oliguria and 12% needing renal replacement therapy. The authors had two conflicting conclusions: (1) that although all of the case subjects had acute kidney injury, "most could not be considered to have contrast nephropathy, since other risk factors for renal failure (both comorbid and iatrogenic) were present" and, that (2) acute kidney injury in this setting is directly associated with increased mortality.[31]

Cause-and-Effect Relationships

That CIN may be a marker for increased mortality risk rather than a contributing cause of death is reviewed by Rudnick and Feldman.[30] These authors performed a literature review that focused on observational studies that assessed factors associated with mortality in patients with CIN, most of which were derived from the cardiac catheterization literature. The observational studies assessed demonstrated that short- and long-term mortality is increased in patients who develop CIN. Most of these studies assessed the relationship between CIN and "downstream" events of morbidity and mortality, which clearly demonstrated that patients experiencing CIN had greater levels of comorbidities at the time of CM administration than patients who did not experience CIN. Independent predictors of in-hospital mortality included age, congestive heart failure, emergent procedures, multivessel procedures, pre-procedural shock, peripheral vascular disease, intra-aortic balloon pump, non-Q-wave infarction, creatine kinase-MB fraction, liver disease, and others. This raises the question of whether these multiple comorbidities are independent causes of death and whether CIN is a contributing factor, or simply a marker. More importantly, putative mechanisms for how CIN is able to cause death or other serious complications have not been elucidated.

A very specific differential between CE-MDCT and percutaneous coronary intervention is the peri-procedural catheterization with coronary intervention versus the noninvasive administration of contrast material with CT.[27] Specifically, with coronary intervention there is a known risk of clot formation during the catheterization procedure, itself, and the possibility of the dislodgement of atheroemboli by the catheter manipulation events necessitated by the procedure itself.[32] Cholesterol emboli are a known cause of acute renal failure.[33]

RANDOM VARIATION

Rao and Newhouse[34] recently highlighted studies performed by Cramer and colleagues[35] and Heller and colleagues[36] because these investigations were the only studies involving patients who received intravenous CM in which control groups of patients who received no CM were reported on. These studies were identified from a MEDLINE database search for articles on CIN and CM in general published between October 1966 and September 2004.[33] This search yielded 3081 publications, 40 of which were found to have reports of renal function in humans after intravenous CM administration. In only 2 of these 40 studies was the incidence of postcontrast renal dysfunction compared with the incidence of renal dysfunction in a matched control group of patients who did not receive CM.

Cramer and colleagues[35] assessed SCr levels before and 2 days after CM-enhanced brain CT in 1993 patients and after nonenhanced brain CT in 233 control patients. A high-osmolality CM (HOCM) (with four to seven times the osmolality of plasma) was administered (60–350 mL). Renal dysfunction following CT, defined as an increase in SCr to greater than 106.1 μmol/L (1.2 mg/dL) and to a level at least 50% higher than the baseline value, developed in four (2.1%) patients in whom CM was infused and in three (1.3%) who received no CM. The difference in renal dysfunction was not significant ($P \geq .05$). In the Cramer and colleagues study,[35] CIN occurred in none of the 19 patients with preexisting renal insufficiency who received HOCM and in 2 (4.3%) of the 46 patients with preexisting renal insufficiency who received no CM (Table 3). Note that to be counted as a case of CIN in their study, one has to have an at least 50% increase in SCr, which is a more stringent criterion than that used by many other authors. In addition, there may have been a lack of comparability between the control patients and those who received CM because the decision to perform unenhanced CT in them may have been based partly on the perceived risk of CIN.

Heller and colleagues[36] examined 292 inpatients who received HOCM and 405 patients who did not receive CM. They also examined a group of patients who received an LOCM, which has two to two and a half times the osmolality of plasma. Patients in the no-contrast-material group were selected on the basis of increased risk of CIN. As such, the low rate of CIN in the HOCM group was partly because of negative selection (selective use in low-risk patients) and the high rate of CIN in the LOCM group was partly because of positive selection (selective use in high-risk patients). Renal impairment was defined as a maximal increase in SCr of 50% or more or of greater than 0.5 mg/dL from the baseline value on at least 1 of the subsequent 4 days. Such outcomes are open to ascertainment bias, as more frequent monitoring in the higher-risk subjects will reveal more cases. CIN was seen in 187 patients who received LOCM, and 23 (12%) of these subjects developed CIN.

In the Heller and colleagues[36] study, an acute increase in SCr was seen in 7 (10%) of 68 patients with preexisting renal insufficiency who received CM versus in 6 (7%) of 88 with preexisting renal insufficiency who did not (see Table 3). It is possible that in any series of ill patients, some will experience renal failure as a coincident event or as an adverse reaction to medication intake or some other nephrotoxic event. There is also the possibility of random variation or "background noise" in the SCr. Another interesting observation

from the Heller and colleagues[36] study was that blood transfusion was an important independent predictor of acute renal failure. This finding highlights the importance of prerenal factors, such as hypotension as a result of to blood loss, and the distinct possibility that CM-induced hypovolemia secondary to nonspecific osmotic diuresis could contribute to CIN in some cases.

Newhouse and colleagues[37] attempted to investigate whether increases in serum creatinine following IV contrast administration constitute random events that occur with a frequency that is similar in patients who do not receive intravenous contrast. In this study, they concluded that fluctuations in serum creatinine levels occur to a similar extent and degree in patients who do not receive intravenous contrast. In 32,161 patients with a serum creatinine drawn for 5 consecutive days who did not undergo contrast administration for 10 days preceding the available creatinine level or during the 5 days of observation, the average creatinine level was 1.65 mg/dL at baseline. Of patients with a baseline creatinine of 0.6 mg/dL or higher, 24% had a change in creatinine level that would have resulted in a diagnosis of "CIN" (defined as a change of at least 25% from baseline) if contrast material had been administered. In patients with a baseline creatinine of 0.6 to 1.2 mg/dL, increases of 25%, 33%, and 50% occurred in 27%, 19%, and 11% respectively. Increases of 0.4, 0.6, and 1.0 mg/dL occurred in 13%, 7%, and 3% of patients. Among patients with baseline creatinine levels greater than 2.0 mg/dL, increases of at least 25%, 33%, and 50% occurred in 16%, 12%, and 7%. Increases of 0.4, 0.6, and 1.0 mg/dL occurred in 33%, 26%, and 18%. To further validate their hypothesis, the authors compared their results with respect to the percentage of random serum creatinine increases with 19 published series of patients who received IV contrast material and were evaluated for a postcontrast creatinine increase. The

Table 3				

Controls with renal insufficiency				
Study	Agents	Prospective	Def CIN	Rates
Cramer et al	HOCM	Yes	↑ SCr ≥ 50%	0% (0/19)
	Controls		↑ SCr ≥ 50%	4.3% (2/46)
Heller et al	HOCM	Yes	↑ SCr ≥ 50%	10% (7/68)
	Controls		↑ SCr ≥ 50%	7% (6/88)
TOTALS	HOCM			8.3% (7/84)
	Controls			5.9% (8/134)

Abbreviations: CIN, contrast-inhanced nephrotoxicity; HOCM, high osmolar contrast media; SCr, serum creatinine.

authors' opinion was that the random increases observed in their study were not different from the incidences of CIN previously published. In all but 5 of these 19 series, the postcontrast serum creatinine increase (absolute value of 0.2–1.0 mg/dL and percentage increase of 25%–50%) was less than the random increases reported by Newhouse and colleagues.[37] Three of those five studies had significant postcontrast creatinine increases (55%–76%); however, patients in these series had renal failure, diabetes, or initial serum creatinine higher than 2.0 mg/dL.

The results of this study suggest that significant changes in creatinine occur in sick patients who do not receive iodinated contrast. The authors concluded that without an appropriate control group, previously published series may not have accurately detected the incidence of CIN (or lack thereof).[37–42] However, the presence of CIN cannot be definitively discounted based on these data because there is not a matched control group of patients who did receive contrast media. Furthermore, there is the risk of selection bias because these subjects had SCr levels measured over several consecutive days suggesting a cohort at greater risk for renal dysfunction or instability than whom such frequent SCr determinations were unnecessary. In spite of these limitations, this study makes clear that there were significant variations in SCr whether or not contrast material was administered.

Bruce and colleagues[42] undertook a retrospective analysis of 11,588 patients undergoing CT (both contrast enhanced and unenhanced) over a 7-year period resulting in 13,274 patient encounters. Patients undergoing CT received either LOCM (iohexol) or IOCM (iodixanol). CIN was defined as an increase in serum creatinine concentration of at least 0.5 mg/dL or a 25% or greater decrease in estimated GFR.

The authors found no significant difference in the overall incidence of CIN between the IOCM contrast (average 8.2%; range 0.0%–18.5%) and control groups (5.9%; 1.3%–9.0%) for all baseline creatinine values.[42] The overall incidence of CIN in the LOCM contrast group (2.1%–10.4%) paralleled that of the control group (1.3%–8.6%) up to a serum creatinine level of 1.8 mg/dL. Increases above this level were associated with a higher incidence of AKI in the LOCM group. Interestingly, the incidence of CIN increased with increasing baseline creatinine concentrations in all three groups, including those not receiving contrast material. The authors concluded that creatinine elevations occur even in patients not receiving contrast during CT examinations, and the risk of CIN may be overstated. They suggest that much of the creatinine elevation in these patients is attributable to background fluctuation, underlying disease, or treatment.

To our knowledge, this is the largest evaluation to date of the incidence of AKI in a control population receiving no contrast material in comparison with a population receiving contrast agent. However, this is also a retrospective nonrandomized study. Such a design may have excluded a large number of cases and introduced a selection bias for patients who presumably had clinical reasons for having their serum creatinine concentration followed. However, and as noted above for the Newhouse and colleagues[37] study, large background fluctuations in SCr are common and have been rarely taken into consideration in assessing the true rates of CIN.[42]

STRATIFICATION OF RISK AND WHAT METRIC?

As for a better understanding of the overall rates of CIN for the intravenous use of CM, there is a growing but still small database that provides some further insight into the question of stratification of risk. By this we mean whether there is a threshold or level of renal function at which the rate of CIN is a much greater risk. Table 4 provides a continually growing overview of the recent data from the prospective assessments of patients at risk with RI and the data having been acquired prospectively. This is an expansion of the information provided in Table 1. Tepel and colleagues[19] studied 42 patients with RI of whom 12 had precontrast material administration SCr of 2.5 mg/dL or greater and 42% (5/12) of these developed CIN. Barrett and colleagues[22] studied 153 subjects with renal insufficiency and had an overall CIN rate of 1.3%. Of those subjects with an SCr of 2.0 mg/dL or greater and with the definition of CIN being an increase of 0.5 mg/dL, observed that 11.1% (2/18) developed CIN. Thomsen and colleagues[23] studied 148 subjects with RI and found an overall CIN rate of 3.4%; whereas in those subjects with SCr of 2.0 mg/dL or greater and/or an eGFR less than or equal to 40 mL/min and criterion for CIN of 0.5 mg/dL observed a rate of CIN of 5.5% (4/73). Kuhn and colleagues[24] studied 248 subjects with RI, finding overall CIN rates of 5.2%. In those patients stratified to have SCr of 2.0 mg/dL or higher, 0% (0/21) developed CIN. In those patients with an eGFR less than or equal to 40 mL/min and with a criterion for CIN of SCr of 25% or greater, observed that 4.8% (1/21) developed CIN. Nguyen and colleagues[20] studied 117 patients with RI and found overall CIN rates of 11.1% but did not stratify for greater degrees of renal insufficiency.

Table 4
Stratification of risk for CIN

Study	All with RI	CIN Rates Overall (%)	Stratification (Criterion)	CIN Rates
Tepel et al (2000)	42	12	SCr ≥2.5 mg/dL (0.5 mg/dL)	42% (5/12)
Barrett et al (2006)	153	1.3	SCr ≥2.0 mg/dL (0.5 mg/dL)	11.1% (2/18)
Thomsen et al (2008)	148	3.4	SCr ≥2.0 mg/dL and/or eGFR ≤40 mL/min (0.5 mg/dL)	5.5% (4/73)
Kuhn et al (2008)	248	5.2	SCr ≥2.0 mg/dL eGFR ≤ 40 mL/min (SCr ≥25%)	0% (0/21) 4.8% (1/21)
Nguyen et al (2008)	117	11.1	Did not stratify	—
Weisbord et al (2008)	367	3.5	eGFR ≤45 mL/min (↑SCr ≥0.5 mg/dL) (↑SCr ≥ 25%)	9.8% (5/51) 11.8% (6/51)

Abbreviations: CIN, contrast-inhanced nephrotoxicity; eGFR, estimated glomerular filtration rate; RI, renal insufficiency; SCr, serum creatinine.

Weisbord and colleagues[21] studied 367 subjects with renal insufficiency and found an overall CIN rate of 3.5% and stratified patients with an eGFR less than or equal to 45 mL/min and an increase in SCr of 0.5 mg/dL or higher observed a 9.8% rate of CIN and using the criterion of an increase in SCr of 25% or more observed an 11.8% rate of CIN.

Overall, these data would appear to suggest that there may be a threshold in patients having a serum creatinine of 2.0 mg/dL or more or an eGFR of less than 40 to 45 mL/min rate of CIN. However, none of these subjects, even with higher stratification of renal dysfunction, required dialysis or died as the result of CIN. Additionally, there is the well-known nonlinear relationship between renal function and SCr especially at the greater stages of RI, which is exactly the subset of subjects that is being presented. Thus, relatively small changes in GFR in these subjects would be manifested by exaggerated changes in serum creatinine or the percentage change in serum creatinine. This has been suggested to represent a potential artifact causing an overrating of CIN with worsening baseline RI.

Of increasing importance is the most appropriate metric for an estimation of baseline renal function and how to rate the relative changes in renal function after the administration of CM. This poses a limitation on how to assess the preexisting clinical data with new studies, as most of the prior studies have used SCr as the baseline metric rather than eGFR. Is it appropriate to adopt the eGFR metric?

The eGFR was established in 1999 and is described by Levey and colleagues in the *Annals of Internal Medicine*.[43,44] The Modification of the Diet in Renal Disease (MDRD) study equation was developed with the use of data from 1628 patients with chronic kidney disease. Ninety-one percent of the GFR estimates were within 30% of the measured values. The GFR standard was the 24-hour renal clearance of ^{125}I-Iothalamate and the equation is derived from a regression analysis that uses SCr, age, gender, and race as the variables. However, there are notable limitations. Importantly, this metric is inaccurate for patients who are not in a study state (such as patients developing acute renal failure). The equation has not been tested in the following subgroups: elderly patients 70 years of age or older; type 1 and type 2 diabetic patients on insulin; patients "with serious comorbid conditions"; transplant recipients; and persons without renal disease. The last limitation is significant since it is exactly those patients who may have borderline renal function that determines the real value for the eGFR, especially patients at the age of 60 or older.

Logistic problems may also arise in that Herts and colleagues found that overall about 6% of patients having CE-MDCT have an SCr greater than or equal to 1.5 mg/dL, whereas the numbers of patient qualifying for "renal insufficiency using the MDRD equation" (eGFR <60 mL/min/1.73 m^2) is 15.3%.[45]

Our overall recommendation is to suggest a liberalization of the criteria for risk threshold at baseline SCr 2.0 mg/dL or greater or an eGFR of less than or equal to 45 mL/min. The recommended approach by the ACR version 6.0 manual on contrast media advises closest attention to patients with chronic kidney disease stages 4 or

5 (eGFR <30 mL/min/1.73 m^2) and not being on chronic dialysis.[46] Patients already on dialysis have no residual renal function to lose and are being adequately managed. However, patients with very poor renal function not on dialysis or patients on intermittent dialysis are at serious risk for progressive renal damage and with no reserve. In these subjects it is prudent to exercise every effort to provide alternative imaging approaches that do not use any type of contrast material. Ultimately, however, clinical exigencies occurring by withholding the contrasted examination must be balanced with the risk of CIN.

PRACTICAL APPROACHES TO REDUCE RISK OF CONTRAST-INDUCED NEPHROTOXICITY

The pathophysiological mechanisms leading to CIN are generally thought to be, alone or in combination, a decrease in renal perfusion, direct CM tabular cell toxicity and free radical formation.[13] Flowing from these concepts are suggestions for prevention. Drugs used in clinical trials to mitigate against the hemodynamic effects have included fenoldopam, theophylline, calcium channel blockers, atrial natruretic peptide, prostaglandin E, and endothelin antagonist, none of which have proved successful. This is further supporting evidence that contrast-induced vasoconstriction is not the major factor. However, there is evidence that hydration to correct pre-renal hypoperfusion is effective.

Strategies to decrease direct cell toxicity have included increasing tubular fluid flow with saline, sodium bicarbonate, or diuretics. Decreasing free radical formation and thus renal injury is by either N-acetylcysteine or sodium bicarbonate infusion.

A detailed discussion of each of the prior studies employing these strategies is beyond the scope of this article and one is encouraged to read the excellent reviews by Mueller[47] Briguori and Marenzi.[48] This topic is also covered elsewhere in this issue of the journal.

Recommendations

Patients considered to be potentially at risk for CIN have an estimated GFR below 60 mL/min. The ACR recommended indications for SCr measurement before intravascular administration of iodinated contrast media include a history of kidney disease, family history of kidney failure, diabetes on medical therapy, paraproteinemia syndromes such as myeloma, collagen vascular disease, prior renal surgery, metformin-containing drug combinations, and treatment with nephrotoxic drugs such as nonsteroidal anti-inflammatory drugs and aminoglycosides.[45] We recommend that all patients should be encouraged to drink water liberally 12 hours before and after contrast exposure when possible.

In elective in-hospital patients, a 24-hour protocol with 1 mL/kg/h saline begun 12 hours before and after the procedure should be implemented. If the contrasted study is emergent, a high rate of 300 mL/h saline 60 minutes before the procedure and continuing for at least 6 hours postcontrast administration is recommended.[47]

SUMMARY

Viewed from multiple perspectives, it appears that there has been an exaggerated emphasis on the morbidity of CIN. Beyond this, a prudent approach for all patients receiving IV CM is adequate hydration pre- and post-imaging. Imaging examinations of clinical necessity should not be withheld for the fear of CIN, however, greater caution is sensible for patients with severe RI where alternative imaging techniques that do not require CM should be seriously considered.

REFERENCES

1. Bartels ED, Baun GC, Gammeltoft A, et al. Acute anuria following intravenous pyelography in a patient with myelomatosis. Acta Med Scand 1954;150: 297–302.
2. Mudge GH. Nephrotoxicity of urographic radiocontrast drugs. Kidney Int 1980;18:540–52.
3. McClennan BL. Ionic and nonionic iodinated contrast media: evolution and strategies for use. Am J Roentgenol 1990;155:225–33.
4. Morris TW. X-ray contrast media: where are we now and where are we going? Radiology 1993;188:11–6.
5. Eloy R, Corot C, Belleville J. Contrast media for angiography: physiochemical properties, pharmacokinetics and biocompatibility. Clin Mater 1991;7:89–97.
6. Katzberg RW. State of the art. Urography into the 21st century: new contrast media, renal handling, imaging characteristics, and nephrotoxicity. Radiology 1997;204:297–312.
7. Stacul F. Current iodinated contrast media. Eur Radiol 2001;11:690–7.
8. Idée J-M, Pinès E, Prigent P, et al. Allergy-like reactions to iodinated contrast agents. A critical analysis. Fundam Clin Pharmacol 2005;19:263–81.
9. Katayama H, Yamaguci K, Kozuka T, et al. Adverse reactions to ionic and nonionic contrast media. A report from the Japanese Committee on Safety of Contrast Media. Radiology 1990;175:621–8.
10. Katzberg RW, Haller C. Contast-induced nephrotoxicity: clinical landscape. Kidney Int 2006;69:53–7.
11. Mudge GH. The maximum urinary concentration of diatrizoates. Invest Radiol 1980;15(Suppl):S67–78.

12. Morris TW, Katzberg RW. Intravascular contrast media: properties and general effects. In: Katzberg RW, editor. The contrast media manual. Baltimore (MD): Williams & Wilkins; 1992. p. 1–18.

13. Katzberg RW. Contrast medium-induced nephrotoxicity: which pathway? [Editorial]. Radiology 2005; 235:752–5.

14. Weisberg LS, Kurnik PB, Kurnik BR. Radiocontrast-induced nephropathy in humans: role of renal vaso-constriction. Kidney Int 1992;41:1408–15.

15. Guevera M, Fernández-Esparrach G, Allessandra C, et al. Effects of contrast media on renal function in patients with cirrhosis: a prospective study. Hepatology 2004;40:646–51.

16. Agmon Y, Peleg H, Greenfeld Z, et al. Nitric oxide and prostanoids protect the renal outer medulla from radiocontrast toxicity in the rat. J Clin Invest 1994;94:1069–75.

17. Lancelot E, Idée JM, Couturier V, et al. Influence of the viscosity of iodixanol on medullary and cortical blood flow in the rat kidney: a potential cause of nephrotoxicity. J Appl Toxicol 1999;19:341–6.

18. Vaamonde CA, Bier RT, Papendick R, et al. Acute and chronic renal effects of radiocontrast in diabetic rats. Role of anesthesia and risk factors. Invest Radiol 1989;24:206–18.

19. Tepel M, van der Geit M, Schwarzfeld C, et al. Prevention of radiocontrast-agent-induced reductions in renal function by acetyleysteine. N Engl J Med 2000;343:180–4.

20. Nguyen SA, Suranyi P, Ravenel JG, et al. Iso-osmolality versus low-osmolality iodinated contrast medium at intravenous contrast-enhanced CT: effect on kidney function. Radiology 2008;248:97–113.

21. Weisbord SD, Mor MK, Resnick AL, et al. Incidence and outcomes of contrast-induced AKI following computed tomography. Clin J Am Soc Nephrol 2008;3:1274–81.

22. Barrett BJ, Katzberg RW, Thomsen HS, et al. Contrast-induced nephropathy in patients with chronic kidney disease undergoing computer tomography. A double blind comparison of iodixanol and iopamidol. Invest Radiol 2006;41:815–21.

23. Thomsen HS, Morcos SK, Earley CM, et al. The ACTIVE trial: comparison of the effects on renal function of iomeprol-400 and iodixanol-320 in patients with chronic kidney disease undergoing abdominal computed tomography. Invest Radiol 2008;43:170–8.

24. Kuhn MJ, Chen N, Sahani DV, et al. The PRDICT study: a randomized double-blind comparison of contrast-induced nephropathy after low- or iso-osmolar contrast agent exposure. Am J Roentgenol 2008;181:151–7.

25. Bellomo R, Kellum JA, Ronco C. Defining and classifying acute renal failure: from advocacy to consensus and validation of RIFLE criteria. Intensive Care Med 2007;33:409–13.

26. Mehta RL, Kellum JA, Shah SV, et al. Acute kidney injury network: report of an initiative to improve outcomes in acute kidney injury. Crit Care 2007;11: 1–8.

27. Katzberg RW, Barrett BJ. Risk of iodinated contrast material-induced nephropathy with intravenous administration. Radiology 2007;243:622–8.

28. Rudnick MR, Goldfarb S, Wexler L, et al. Nephrotoxicity of ionic and nonionic contrast media in 1196 patients: a randomized trial. The Iohexol Cooperative Study. Kidney Int 1995;47(1):254–61.

29. Gruberg L, Mintz GS, Mehran R, et al. The prognostic implications of further renal function deterioration within 48 h of interventional coronary procedures in patients with pre-existent chronic renal insufficiency. J Am Coll Cardiol 2000;36: 1542–8.

30. Rudnick M, Feldman H. Contrast-induced nephropathy: what are the true clinical consequences. Clin J Am Soc Nephrol 2008;3:263–72.

31. Levy EM, Viscoli CM, Horwitz RI. The effect of acute renal failure on mortality: a cohort analysis. JAMA 1996;275:1489–94.

32. Keeley EC, Grines CL. Scraping of aortic debris by coronary guiding catheters. A prospective evolution in 1,000 cases. J Am Coll Cardiol 1998;32(7): 1861–5.

33. Vidt DG. Cholesterol emboli, a common cause of renal failure. Annu Rev Med 1997;48:375–85.

34. Rao Q, Newhouse JH. Risk of nephropathy after intravenous contrast: a critical literature analysis. Radiology 2006;239:392–7.

35. Cramer BC, Parfrey PS, Hutchinson TA, et al. Renal function following infusion of radiologic contrast material: a prospective controlled study. Arch Intern Med 1985;145:87–9.

36. Heller CA, Knapp J, Halliday J, et al. Failure to demonstrate contrast nephrotoxicity. Med J Aust 1991;155:329–32.

37. Newhouse JH, Kho D, Rao QA, et al. Frequency of serum creatinine charges in the absence of iodinated contrast material: implications for studies of contrast nephrotoxicity. Am J Roentgenol 2008; 191:376–82.

38. Shafi T, Chon SY, Porush JG, et al. Infusion intravenous pyelography and renal function: effects in patients with chronic renal insufficiency. Arch Intern Med 1978;138:1218–21.

39. Harkonen S, Kjellstrand CM. Exacerbation of diabetic renal failure following intravenous pyelography. Am J Med 1977;63(6):939–46.

40. Smith HJ, Levorstad K, Berg KJ, et al. High dose urography in patients with renal failure: a double-blind investigation of iohexol and metrizoate. Acta Radiol Diagn 1985;26:213–20.

41. Teruel JL, Marcen R, Onaindia JM, et al. Renal function impairment caused by intravenous urography: a

prospective study. Arch Intern Med 1981;141: 1271–4.

42. Bruce RJ, Djamali A, Shinki K, et al. Background fluctuation of kidney function versus contrast-induced nephrotoxicity. Am J Roentgenol 2009; 192:711–8.

43. Levey AS, Bosch JP, Lewis JB, et al. A more accurate method to estimate glomerular filtration rate from serum creatinine: a new prediction equation. Modification of diet in renal disease study group. Ann Intern Med 1999;130:461–70.

44. Levey AS, Coresh J, Balk E, et al. National kidney foundation practice guidelines for chronic kidney disease: evolution, classification, and stratification. Ann Intern Med 2003;139:137–47.

45. Herts BR, Schneider E, Poggio ED, et al. Identifying outpatients with renal insufficiency before contrast-enhanced CT by using estimated glomerular filtration rates versus serum creatinine levels. Radiology 2008;248:106–13.

46. American College of Radiology Manual on Contrast Media, version 6.0. American College of Radiology website, Available at: http://www.acr.org. Accessed March 8, 2009.

47. Mueller C. Prevention of contrast-induced nephropathy with volume supplementation. Kidney Int Suppl 2006;100:S16–9.

48. Briguori C, Marenzi G. Contrast-induced nephropathy: pharmacological prophylaxis. Kidney Int 2006;69:530–8.

Prevention of Contrast-Induced Nephropathy: An Overview

James H. Ellis, MD*, Richard H. Cohan, MD

KEYWORDS

- Iodinated contrast material • Nephropathy
- Nephrotoxicity • Contrast-induced nephropathy
- Prevention • Renal function

In recent years, contrast-induced nephropathy (CIN) has become an increasingly controversial subject, even as newer low-osmolality contrast media (LOCM) and iso-osmolality contrast media (ICM) have reduced the risk[1,2] compared with previously used high-osmolality contrast media (HOCM). On one front, controversy has arisen over the validity of much of the scientific literature on CIN, which has been challenged based on the absence of control groups that did not receive contrast media.[3–5] On the other front, continuing efforts to find ways to prevent the occurrence of CIN have themselves generated controversy over the efficacy of the individual approaches. This article addresses the controversies surrounding the many attempts to solve the issue of CIN by preventing it from occurring.

One of the difficulties in assessing methods to reduce the risk of CIN is that all interventions that attempt to reduce CIN risk have risks themselves. Fortunately, most are low-risk interventions. The risk of developing CIN and its consequences are beyond the scope of this review. Nevertheless, the reader is cautioned to place those risks in perspective with the hazards entailed by using CIN-preventive maneuvers; these will vary from patient to patient, making the decision-making process more difficult. Furthermore, even if it is true that patients who develop CIN have more clinical adverse events than patients who do not develop CIN (as suggested by many[6–9] but not all[10] studies), it remains to be proven that CIN is the cause of those adverse outcomes or that preventing CIN would reduce the number of adverse outcomes. It is possible that the development of CIN is simply an indicator for patients who would fare poorly under any circumstances.

METHODS TO REDUCE THE RISK OF CONTRAST-INDUCED NEPHROPATHY
Dose Reduction or Elimination

The risk of CIN can be completely avoided by obtaining the required diagnostic information using tests that do not require the intravascular administration of radiographic iodinated contrast media (RICM). For example, it may be possible to substitute ultrasound, noncontrast CT, or noncontrast MR for a contrast-enhanced CT study. Clearly the use of noncontrast CT for evaluation of urinary tract stone disease has markedly reduced the number of RICM administrations for excretory urography.[11]

In some cases, it may not be reasonable to omit RICM entirely, but it may be possible to use a lower dose than usual as the renal toxicity of RICM is dose-dependent.[12] For example, a substantial portion of the RICM dose in abdominopelvic CT is administered to opacify the liver parenchyma.[13,14] If optimum hepatic parenchymal opacification is not necessary, such as in a search for a postoperative intra-abdominal abscess, the dose may be reduced. Care should be taken that the amount is not reduced so much that

Department of Radiology, University of Michigan Health System, B1-D502 University Hospital, SPC 5030, 1500 E. Medical Center Drive, Ann Arbor, Michigan 48109-5030, USA
* Corresponding author.
E-mail address: jimellis@umich.edu (J.H. Ellis).

Radiol Clin N Am 47 (2009) 801–811
doi:10.1016/j.rcl.2009.06.003
0033-8389/09/$ – see front matter © 2009 Elsevier Inc. All rights reserved.

a nondiagnostic study is obtained, yet the patient is exposed to the CIN risk of the RICM given.

For studies in which RICM is injected to directly opacify an artery or vein, it may be possible to use carbon dioxide as the contrast agent instead because it has a low risk of nephrotoxicity.[15–19] It has also been suggested that carbon dioxide use can be supplemented with injections of gadolinium-based contrast material (GBCM)[16,19] or RICM.[17–19] In the latter instance, lesser amounts of RICM are required when carbon dioxide is used. However, the use of GBCM alone or in combination with carbon dioxide in preference to RICM for radiographic examinations is not recommended in patients with reduced renal function because equi-attenuating amounts of gadolinium-based contrast agents are potentially more nephrotoxic than RICM.[20] In addition, the recent association between certain types of GBCM and nephrogenic systemic fibrosis (NSF) in patients with marked renal dysfunction inhibits the utility of the combined carbon dioxide-GBCM approach. The use of carbon dioxide for angiography is covered in more detail elsewhere in this issue.

Choice of Specific Radiographic Iodinated Contrast Media

One of the advantages of LOCM over HOCM is its reduced rate of CIN in at-risk patients.[21] The underlying reason for this reduced CIN risk has not been clearly established. Potential explanations include reduced osmolality, different ionicity, and/or other physiochemical properties.[22] If the risk reduction were attributable to reduced osmolality, it would be reasonable to test whether the even lower osmolality of ICM might lead to a further reduction in risk.

Whether some iso- or low-osmolality iodinated contrast agents are more or less nephrotoxic than others has become an enormous controversy, even spurring litigation over claims of false advertising.[23] One question that can be raised is whether CIN risk might be reduced by using the iso-osmolality agent iodixanol (Visipaque; GE Healthcare, Princeton, NJ). Over three dozen studies have sought to determine if intravascular iodixanol is less nephrotoxic than various LOCM that have been used for comparison.[24] Some studies have shown no difference, some have shown that iodixanol use resulted in a reduced rate of CIN, and some have shown that iodixanol use resulted in an increased rate of CIN. Two meta-analyses[22,24] of these CIN studies have been performed, and they came to opposite conclusions. The lack of uniformity in the results of these studies has led to a second question:

whether there might be a range of CIN risk over which the entire armamentarium of iso- and low-osmolality RICM might be distributed.[25] It is at least conceivable that iodixanol might fall somewhere in the middle of CIN risk for all of the lower osmolality RICM. Such behavior could explain the differing results of the various studies of iodixanol and CIN.

The meta-analysis of McCullough and colleagues[22] examined studies of angiographic examinations in which CIN was defined as a rise in serum creatinine (SCr) of 0.5 mg/dL or greater. In this meta-analysis, iodixanol showed a lower CIN risk than the pooled comparator LOCM for patients who had chronic kidney disease (defined as baseline SCr of 1.5 mg/dL or greater for men or 1.3 mg/dL or greater for women, or baseline creatinine clearance of 60 mL/min or less). No statistically significant difference in risk was present for patients who did not have chronic kidney disease. Of the 1345 patients in the LOCM group, 789 (59%) received ioxaglate (Hexabrix; Covidien, St. Louis, MO), 381 (28%) received iohexol (Omnipaque; GE Healthcare), and 175 (13%) received iopromide (Ultravist; Bayer HealthCare Pharmaceuticals, Wayne, NJ) or iopamidol (Isovue; Bracco Diagnostics, Princeton, NJ). The dose of the contrast agent was significantly ($P = .003$) higher in the LOCM examinations (mean of 58.9 g I) in comparison to the iodixanol examinations (mean of 55.4 g I). The meta-analysis of Heinrich and colleagues[24] included studies of intravenous administration of RICM as well as studies of intra-arterial RICM administration, but the meta-analysis excluded studies where ioxaglate was the comparator. CIN was defined either as an SCr increase of 0.5 mg/dL or greater, or as an SCr increase of 25% or greater. In this meta-analysis, no significant difference was observed in the risk of CIN between iodixanol and the pooled LOCM. However, in a subgroup analysis, iodixanol use did demonstrate lower CIN rates than iohexol use for intra-arterial administration in patients with renal insufficiency (renal insufficiency was variably defined by the individual studies analyzed). In none of the seven included studies of intravenous injection was a difference in risk reported.

The results of these two studies demonstrate that meta-analyses cannot be relied on as sources of truth. If that were so, they could not differ in their conclusions. Meta-analyses may be limited by the validity of the studies they include for review, and the heterogeneity of the results. Furthermore, many of the individual studies analyzed within the aforementioned meta-analyses can be criticized on methodological grounds. Relative CIN risk among RICM is an issue that would be best pursued by a large well-designed randomized trial among multiple agents, rather than by meta-analyses of potentially heterogeneous studies that compare only two agents to each other. However, given the variation in serum creatinine in ill patients who do not receive RICM,[4] it will be difficult to complete a study that accurately assesses the low CIN risk of RICM on this background noise of "hospital-induced nephropathy."[5] It seems likely that any differences between RICM, even if real, will be small.

We believe that at the present time, it is difficult to discern a clear CIN advantage for ICM for intravenous use, and that it is reasonable to use either LOCM or ICM once the decision to administer RICM intravenously has been made (that is, once it has been decided that the potential benefits of RICM administration outweigh the potential risks). There is limited evidence[22,24] that for intra-arterial administration there may be a lessened CIN risk, of uncertain importance, for iodixanol compared with iohexol and ioxaglate in patients with preexisting renal dysfunction. There is insufficient evidence to determine a specific threshold of renal dysfunction at which the substitution of ICM for LOCM should be made. Most importantly, however, one should not assume that substitution of ICM for LOCM is by itself a sufficient precaution in every at-risk patient. All RICM present some CIN risk, albeit low for clinically consequential nephropathy.

Hydration

Hydration is the intervention that has most consistently been demonstrated effective in reducing the risk of CIN.[12,26–28] Its advantages include low cost and low risk to the patient in all but the most fluid-intolerant patients. There is a presumptive physiologic explanation for why hydration may reduce the risk of CIN: properly performed, hydration increases intravascular volume and induces diuresis causing dilution of the RICM in the renal tubules and decreasing the contact time within the kidney. Diuresis also leads to vasodilatation in the vulnerable region of the renal medulla possibly through increasing the production of prostacycline. In addition, volume expansion suppresses the renin-angiotensin system and the production of the antidiuretic hormone (ADH), both of which induce renal vasoconstriction. However, it is conceivable that hydration may also dilute (ie, lower) SCr, resulting in a smaller apparent rise in SCr in hydrated patients compared with nonhydrated patients, and making hydration appear to be more protective against CIN than it really is. Indeed, in a study[29] designed to determine the renal effects of iopentol, a control group that received intravenous normal saline showed a statistically significant decrease in SCr measured 3 hours after the saline was administered. Nonetheless, it seems unlikely that the diluting effect of hydration on serum creatinine would persist for more than a few hours after the stoppage of the fluid administration in most cases, although the duration might be prolonged in the presence of low urine output. Regardless, the use of hydration is so widely accepted that it has become routine and is essentially the standard against which other maneuvers are compared for CIN prevention in at-risk patients.

Hydration may be given intravenously or orally. Some studies indicate that intravenous hydration more effectively reduces the risk of CIN than oral hydration alone.[26] For intravenous hydration, Mueller and colleagues[27] showed that using normal saline was more effective than using half-normal saline. Intravenous administration of a 154 mEq/L solution of sodium bicarbonate has been proposed as an effective method of hydration that is superior to normal saline in reducing CIN risk,[30] presumably because of its alkalizing properties. However, other studies have shown sodium bicarbonate infusion to be no more effective than saline infusion[31] or even less effective.[6] Reviews and meta-analyses have noted that the evidence regarding sodium bicarbonate hydration is mixed.[26,32–34] It is possible that publication bias favoring positive results might contribute to early enthusiasm for sodium bicarbonate hydration. Additional studies will be required to resolve this issue definitively. Until then, there is little reason to choose either sodium bicarbonate or saline hydration over the other.

Unfortunately, neither the optimum nor the minimum effective timing and duration of intravenous or oral hydration are known. Beginning earlier and continuing longer is probably better.[26–28] Sample intravenous regimens include 2 mL/kg body weight for 2 hours before RICM administration and 1 mL/kg during and for 6 hours after the procedure,[31] and 1 mL/kg for 12 hours before through 12 hours after the procedure.[35] These hydration protocols were designed for patients undergoing cardiac and arteriographic procedures. Indeed most studies of CIN involve arteriographic examinations. These hydration protocols would be inconvenient for most RICM administrations, which are intravenous for outpatient CT. Fortunately, the incidence of CIN following intravenous RICM is low and often alternative imaging is available for patients at the highest risk. Preliminary evidence[36] has suggested that 2 days of oral sodium chloride (given in capsules) might result in a similar CIN risk as a 6-hour pre-procedure regimen of intravenous normal saline; the use of oral sodium chloride may result in extracellular volume expansion that oral water does not provide.[28] The statistical power of this study has been questioned.[28,36] More investigation will be required before assuming the equivalency of oral and intravenous hydration regimens.

Pharmaceutical Premedication

Premedicating the patient before RICM injection with a pharmaceutical that prevents CIN is the "holy grail" of those who administer RICM. Despite years of searching, no perfect drug to prevent CIN has yet been discovered.

One instructive experience is the rise and fall of the use of fenoldopam (Corlopam; Abbott Laboratories, Abbott Park, IL) for preventing CIN. Fenoldopam is a selective dopamine-1-receptor agonist for intravenous use as an antihypertensive. In 2001, Madyoon and colleagues[37] published a study of 46 patients with SCr above 1.4 mg/dL who underwent angiographic procedures and who received fenoldopam as a continuous intravenous infusion beginning 2 hours before the procedure and continuing for at least 4 hours after. The patients required frequent monitoring to avoid hypotension. CIN was defined as an increase in SCr, compared with baseline, of 25% or more at 48 hours after RICM administration. CIN was observed in 6 (13%) of the 46 patients. The study included no control group. Instead, the rate of CIN was compared with another study in which the rate of CIN was 19 (38%) of 50 patients. The authors stated that they were "very encouraged" by their results and suggested that use of fenoldopam might decrease CIN incidence in azotemic patients; still, they recommended further investigation in randomized controlled trials. Nevertheless, results of this study led to considerable excitement with some institutions adopting this technique. However, by 2003, three randomized placebo-controlled studies of 78,[38] 45,[39] and 315[40] patients had shown no CIN-protective effect of fenoldopam. The fenoldopam experience confirms "the importance of completing adequately powered, prospective, double-blind randomized controlled trials before active therapies are adopted into widespread use."[40]

Fortunately, most other pharmacologic interventions investigated for possible reduction of CIN risk have been tested in controlled studies. However, not all of these studies have been large or multi-institutional, and not all have been replicated before their putative solution has been widely adopted. In 2000, Tepel and colleagues[41] published a study of 83 patients with chronic renal insufficiency undergoing RICM administration and hydrated with intravenous fluids, of which approximately half received oral N-acetylcysteine (NAC, an antioxidant medication) and approximately half received a placebo. Comparing the baseline SCr to one obtained 48 hours after RICM administration, and defining CIN as a rise in SCr of 0.5 mg/dL or greater, Tepel and colleagues[41] found a statistically significant difference in the percentage of control patients (21%, 9 of 42) who met the definition of CIN compared with the patients who were premedicated with NAC (2%, 1 of 41). The day after publication, a patient who had started NAC the day of publication was sent for a contrast-enhanced CT scan at our institution.

Since the publication of Tepel and colleagues,[41] there have been at least 30 additional randomized controlled trials published that have evaluated the efficacy of NAC in reducing the risk of CIN.[42] Some have used oral administration of NAC and in others NAC has been infused intravenously. The results have been mixed. To try to resolve these conflicting results, over a dozen meta-analyses have been performed, also without a clear resolution. In furtherance of the goal of deciding whether NAC protects against CIN, some authors[43–46] have analyzed the meta-analyses. These reviews have shown that the published meta-analyses are rather evenly distributed between those that conclude that NAC is effective in reducing CIN risk and those that conclude that the evidence is insufficient to support NAC use for this purpose. Criticisms of the published meta-analyses include various forms of bias such as publication bias that can limit the utility of meta-analyses[44,45] and the inappropriate aggregation of heterogeneous studies.[43–46] These challenges to the published meta-analyses further weaken the already conflicting evidence supporting the use of NAC to reduce CIN risk.

A challenge to the use of NAC has been raised on the grounds that NAC might lower SCr without truly affecting renal function. In one study,[47] a statistically significant lowering of SCr levels with concomitant rise in estimated glomerular filtration rate (eGFR) occurred in a group of 50 healthy volunteers who received NAC but were not exposed to RICM. Cystatin C, a more accurate estimator of GFR than SCr,[47–49] was measured to determine if the change in SCr might be because of actual improvement in renal function. The cystatin C levels did not change significantly, suggesting that the lowering of SCr was an artifact of NAC administration. In the clinical studies that evaluated the utility of NAC in reducing CIN, it is possible that the patients who received NAC may have experienced similar renal damage as the control patients, but that the NAC may have merely appeared to protect the former from CIN by artificially lowering their SCr, perhaps for only a few days (most studies of CIN follow patients for no more than 72 hours). Credence to this theory has been lent by the study of Poletti and colleagues,[50] in which renal insufficiency patients who received intravenous RICM for CT were randomized to receive NAC or placebo. When CIN was defined using SCr levels, there was a statistically significant difference in the rate of CIN between NAC and placebo groups, but when CIN was defined using cystatin C values, no difference was observed.

The study of Hoffmann and colleagues[47] has been criticized for using normal volunteers with large reserves of renal function who differ from the renal insufficiency patients who clinically receive NAC to protect against CIN. Rehman and colleagues[51] administered oral liquid NAC to chronic kidney disease patients who did not receive RICM, and found no significant changes in SCr or cystatin C. These authors concluded that the alterations in SCr observed in studies of NAC were likely related to true changes in GFR. However, the study of Rehman and colleagues[51] included only 29 patients. Additionally, the potency of the liquid formulation of NAC has been questioned.[52] If liquid oral NAC is not potent, then the absence of changes in SCr and cystatin C in the study of Rehman and colleagues[51] is not good evidence against the theory that NAC may artificially lower SCr.

It is possible that even if NAC artificially lowers SCr, it might still protect kidneys against CIN to some extent. To answer this question, a long-term study would be required, so that patients might be evaluated after the putative direct SCr-lowering effects of NAC had passed. Most studies of NAC do not follow patients longer than about 3 days. However, in one series[10] of percutaneous coronary interventions, patients were followed for 9 months. No statistically significant differences were identified between the NAC and control patients in several relevant clinical measures. NAC did not reduce the frequency of urgent dialysis in this study or when the study's data was combined with that from seven prior NAC studies.

There are studies in the interventional cardiology literature that suggest that, apart from CIN, RICM-exposed patients who receive NAC do better in their general health status during that acute episode of care than patients who do not receive NAC.[9] Other studies have not found this difference.[10] Because NAC is a cardioprotective drug, it is not clear how much of the differences in

outcome, if they exist, are a result of the cardiac versus the renal effects of the drug.[9] Therefore it is possible that NAC may be a useful drug in some situations involving RICM even if it does not protect against CIN.

Overall, it is difficult not to compare the experience with NAC to that previously observed with fenoldopam. Despite the conflicting and unsatisfactory evidence supporting the use of NAC to prevent CIN, and the absence of a definitive study,[52] NAC very quickly has become widely used[52,53] and administration of NAC has been described as the standard of care[53] for reducing CIN risk, even though its efficacy remains unproven.

A number of other drugs have been administered in attempts to reduce the frequency of CIN. In general, these drugs have not consistently demonstrated efficacy in CIN prevention. Furthermore, studies evaluating these agents have lacked a control group that received the drug but did not receive RICM. Such a control group is necessary to demonstrate that the drug itself does not lower SCr. If the drug does lower SCr, then the study must include methods of showing that renal impairment from RICM is actually reduced or prevented by the drug. Otherwise, the drug may simply appear to reduce CIN without actually doing so. Achieving such a control group is difficult; perhaps the best that can be hoped for is a group of matched control patients.

The list of drugs that have been evaluated for the prevention of CIN is long. Some have advocated the use of theophylline, in part because it needs to be administered for only a brief period before RICM administration.[54] However, the data are not conclusive: one meta-analysis[55] found a statistically significant difference in SCr changes for theophylline compared with placebo (but without being able to determine if there was a clinically meaningful benefit), whereas two other meta-analyses did not show statistically significant effects.[42,56] A sampling of tested drugs for which there is even more limited, conflicting, or negative evidence include dopamine,[42] furosemide,[35,42,57] mannitol,[35,42] probucol,[58] ascorbic acid,[42,59] atrial natriuretic peptide,[60] captopril,[61] nifedipine,[62] nitrendipine and other calcium channel blockers,[63] and prostaglandin E1.[64,65] Several recent reviews[66–71] have detailed a wide variety of approaches to preventing CIN, including drug therapies.

Hemodialysis and Hemofiltration

Hemodialysis removes LOCM and ICM from the blood. Several studies have been published testing whether postcontrast hemodialysis might reduce the rate of CIN.[72–74] A systematic review of the literature[72] found that hemodialysis, even when performed as soon as possible after contrast administration, is not effective in reducing the frequency of CIN. This may be because the injury to the kidneys from RICM occurs shortly after it is injected, although even performing hemodialysis concurrently with RICM administration did not show efficacy.[72] Hemodialysis has its own set of risks associated with the procedure, and can in some instances be nephrotoxic because of activation of inflammation and volume depletion.[73]

Hemofiltration is a continuous form of renal replacement therapy. As solutes and water are removed from the bloodstream, the escaping fluids are replaced with large volumes of isotonic fluid, which serves to maintain hemodynamic stability.[67,75] With hemofiltration, some of the RICM is removed from the blood while the remaining RICM is diluted by the isotonic replacement fluid.[76] In a study of 114 patients,[76] the incidence of CIN was reduced substantially in the patients treated with hemofiltration for 4 to 8 hours before the procedure and 18 to 24 hours afterward, in comparison with the patients who received intravenous hydration with normal saline. Subsequently, Marenzi and colleagues[75] determined that hemofiltration must be initiated before RICM administration to be effective. Hemofiltration is an expensive procedure that is performed in the intensive care setting. Although it may eventually prove to be of value in a highly selected patient population at extremely high risk of CIN, the evidence for its efficacy at present remains limited,[71] making it difficult to justify widespread adoption in view of its cost and invasiveness. Furthermore, hemofiltration, like hemodialysis, lowers SCr intrinsically, and thus using SCr as the sole marker of renal injury may be inappropriate. Including other markers of renal function or injury could help distinguish potentially confounding effects of mechanically lowering SCr.[72]

PRACTICAL APPROACH TO REDUCING CONTRAST-INDUCED NEPHROPATHY RISK

Most CIN resolves without untoward clinical effects in the involved patients. Clinically important CIN occurs only occasionally and it is not possible to predict with certainty which patients will suffer from this significant complication of RICM administration. The traditional teaching is that the more severe the patient's baseline renal dysfunction, the more likely it is that the patient will develop CIN, and the more likely that CIN will be clinically significant. However, Newhouse and colleagues[4] showed that those patients with higher SCr at baseline had larger absolute increases in SCr in subsequent determinations, even in the absence of any exposure to RICM. Therefore, a study using a fixed threshold for diagnosing CIN, such as a rise in SCr of 0.5 mg/dL or more, might overestimate the incidence of CIN, unless the study used matched control patients who did not receive RICM. Without this control group, it is not possible to estimate the background changes in SCr that occurred, unrelated to RICM exposure, in the study population. It is also worth emphasizing that studies evaluating the incidence of CIN in patients with reduced renal function should recruit only patients with stable SCr for several weeks before RICM administration to ensure that any further rise in SCr is due to a new acute renal insult caused by the contrast agent and not reflective of progressive deterioration in renal function caused by the primary kidney disease or other factors that influence renal function.

There is no consensus, official or otherwise, among radiologists as to the level of baseline renal dysfunction that raises the risk of clinically significant CIN to the point where intervention should be undertaken.[77] For patients with all levels of renal insufficiency, the radiologist should determine whether using intravascular RICM is in the patient's interest despite the potential CIN risk, and should consider whether an alternate way of obtaining the needed diagnostic information that does not require intravascular RICM use would be a better choice. Given the unknowns about the actual risk of CIN, this is difficult to do with certainty, and so such assessments must be done qualitatively, and somewhat subjectively. On the other hand, patients should not be denied the benefits of RICM administration, when truly beneficial to the patient's care, because of exaggerated fears of CIN. Although not the official position of any scientific body of which we are aware, one recommendation (H.S. Thomsen, presented at the 2008 annual meeting of the Radiological Society of North America) is to take precautions before intra-arterial administration of RICM if the eGFR is less than 60 mL/min and before intravenous administration of RICM if the eGFR is less than 40 mL/min. A pooled analysis[78] of two studies[79,80] of intravenous administration of RICM found that only 1 (0.6%) of 170 patients with eGFR over 40 mL/min experienced a rise in SCR that equaled or exceeded 0.5 mg/dL. The presumed greater risk of CIN from intra-arterial compared with intravenous RICM administration[81] explains the two different thresholds.

Three clinical situations warrant special consideration. No clinically relevant additional damage following RICM administration occurs to the kidneys of an anuric patient with end stage renal disease (ESRD) receiving dialysis. In this group of patients, LOCM or ICM can be used without apprehension, and can be administered without concern for the timing of subsequent dialysis.[82] Anuric ESRD patients must be differentiated from the group of patients who are on permanent dialysis but who have residual renal function and urine production that could be reduced or lost following RICM administration. The latter patients may be among the highest risk patients for clinically relevant CIN, as the urine that they do produce can contribute substantially to a better quality of life over becoming an anuric patient. The third group comprises those patients with acute kidney injury (AKI), regardless of whether or not they are being treated with dialysis. In these patients, both the underlying degree of renal injury and the prospects for recovery may be unknown. Therefore, it is wise not to layer on the additional possibly nephrotoxic intervention of RICM administration unless absolutely necessary. In the latter two of the three special groups discussed, consultation with the referring clinician and the patient may be advisable, and the use of risk reduction strategies may be proper.

SUMMARY

Many unknowns remain about the incidence and significance of CIN, about the efficacy of interventions designed to reduce the risk of CIN, and about the thresholds that indicate when these interventions should be applied (Box 1). Nevertheless, it remains widely accepted that the need to reduce CIN risk increases as the patient's baseline renal function decreases, until the patient's kidneys are completely nonfunctional, at which point CIN risk is no longer pertinent. One recommendation suggests that special precautions, beyond any that might be employed for patients with normal renal function, are not necessary for intravenous RICM administration in patients with an eGFR of 40 mL/min or greater or for intra-arterial RICM administration in patients with an eGFR of 60 mL/min or greater. Patients who fall outside these thresholds or who present with AKI must be evaluated carefully, and imaging studies not requiring RICM injection should be considered. However, there is no absolute renal contraindication to RICM administration should that be absolutely necessary.

Strategies to reduce CIN risk include avoiding the administration of RICM through the use of imaging tests that do not require it, or reducing the dose while still obtaining a diagnostic study.

> **Box 1**
> **Recommendations for the prevention of contrast-induced nephropathy**
>
> Identify patients at risk
>
>   Acute kidney injury
>
>   Chronic renal disease
>
>   eGFR < 40 mL/min for intravenous RICM administration
>
>   eGFR < 60 mL/min for intra-arterial administration
>
>   Risk increases with decreasing renal function
>
>   Exception: ESRD patients with permanently absent renal function are without risk of CIN
>
> Potential precautions in at-risk patients:
>
>   Substitute a test that does not use RICM
>
>   Reduce the dose of RICM while still obtaining a diagnostic study
>
>   For vascular studies, substitute carbon dioxide for some or all of the RICM
>
>   Hydration
>
>   Hemofiltration in exceptional circumstances
>
>   Other precautionary measures are unproven
>
> Evaluate the risks and possible benefits of RICM and potential CIN precautions
>
>   There is no absolute renal contraindication to RICM administration
>
>   Most CIN (if it occurs) resolves without untoward clinical effects, but permanent reduction in renal function can occur in some cases

Hydration remains the most consistently recommended maneuver to reduce CIN risk, and it is inexpensive and, in most patients, is risk free. Other interventions to reduce CIN risk are controversial, with the data often limited by lack of appropriate control groups and publication bias. Many interventions are inconvenient, expensive, or both. Some that held promise at the outset subsequently have proved to be ineffective or even detrimental after definitive studies were performed, and some have their own risks to the patient. None of these other interventions have been conclusively proven to be effective, and therefore it is difficult to recommend them for general use. Although use of the antioxidant NAC is popular, has low risk, and gives the impression of "doing something," its efficacy remains unproven. Whether differences in the oral preparation (solid or liquid), or in the route of administration (oral or intravenous), of NAC make a difference in terms of efficacy remains to be determined. In exceptional circumstances, hemofiltration can be considered for CIN prophylaxis.

ACKNOWLEDGMENT

Both authors are co-investigators without salary in an iodinated contrast media research project sponsored by GE Healthcare, and both authors are consultants to a legal firm representing GE Healthcare related to gadolinium-based contrast media.

REFERENCES[1]

1. Barrett BJ, Carlisle EJ. Metaanalysis of the relative nephrotoxicity of high- and low-osmolality iodinated contrast media. Radiology 1993;188(1):171–8 {A}.

2. Rudnick MR, Goldfarb S, Wexler L, et al. Nephrotoxicity of ionic and nonionic contrast media in 1196 patients: a randomized trial. Kidney Int 1995;47(1):254–61 {A}.

3. Rao QA, Newhouse JH. Risk of nephropathy after intravenous administration of contrast material: a critical literature analysis. Radiology 2006;239(2):392–7 {B}.

4. Newhouse JH, Kho D, Rao QA, et al. Frequency of serum creatinine changes in the absence of iodinated contrast material: implications for studies of contrast nephrotoxicity. AJR Am J Roentgenol 2008;191(2):376–82 {B}.

5. Baumgarten DA, Ellis JH. Contrast-induced nephropathy: contrast material not required? AJR Am J Roentgenol 2008;191(2):383–6.

6. From AM, Bartholmai BJ, Williams AW, et al. Sodium bicarbonate is associated with an increased incidence of contrast nephropathy: a retrospective cohort study of 7977 patients at Mayo Clinic. Clin J Am Soc Nephrol 2008;3(1):10–8 {B}.

7. Brown JR, Malenka DJ, DeVries JT, et al. Transient and persistent renal dysfunction are predictors of survival after percutaneous coronary intervention: insights from the Dartmouth Dynamic Registry. Catheter Cardiovasc Interv 2008;72(3):347–54 {B}.

8. Levy EM, Viscoli CM, Horwitz RI. The effect of acute renal failure on mortality. A cohort analysis. JAMA 1996;275(19):1489–94 {B}.

9. Marenzi G, Assanelli E, Marana I, et al. N-acetyl-cysteine and contrast-induced nephropathy in primary angioplasty. N Engl J Med 2006;354(26):2773–82 {A}.

10. Miner SES, Dzavik V, Nguyen-Ho P, et al. N-acetyl-cysteine reduces contrast-associated nephropathy but not clinical events during long-term follow-up. Am Heart J 2004;148(4):690–5 {A}.

11. Pfister SA, Deckart A, Laschke S, et al. Unenhanced helical computed tomography vs intravenous urography in patients with acute flank pain: accuracy and economic impact in a randomized prospective trial. Eur Radiol 2003;13(11):2513–20 {A}.

12. Committee on Drugs and Contrast Media. Manual on contrast media, version 6. Available at: http://acr.org/SecondaryMainMenuCategories/quality_safety/contrast_manual.aspx. Accessed January 4, 2009.

13. Brink JA. Contrast optimization and scan timing for single and multidetector-row computed tomography. J Comput Assist Tomogr 2003;27(Suppl 1):S3–8.

14. Ichikawa T, Erturk SM, Araki T. Multiphasic contrast-enhanced multidetector-row CT of liver: contrast-enhancement theory and practical scan protocol with a combination of fixed injection duration and patients' body-weight-tailored dose of contrast material. Eur J Radiol 2006;58(2):165–76.

15. Hahn ST, Pfammatter T, Cho KJ. Carbon dioxide gas as a venous contrast agent to guide upper-arm insertion of central venous catheters. Cardiovasc Intervent Radiol 1995;18(3):146–9.

16. Kim H, Tsai J, Paxton B. Safety and utility of uterine artery embolization with CO_2 and a gadolinium-based contrast medium. J Vasc Interv Radiol 2007;18(8):1021–7.

17. Dewald CL, Jensen CC, Park YH, et al. Vena cavography with CO_2 versus with iodinated contrast material for inferior vena cava filter placement: a prospective evaluation. Radiology 2000;216(3):752–7 {A}.

18. Liss P, Eklof H, Hellberg O, et al. Renal effects of CO_2 and iodinated contrast media in patients undergoing renovascular intervention: a prospective, randomized study. J Vasc Interv Radiol 2005;16(1):57–65 {A}.

19. Spinosa DJ, Angle JF, Hagspiel KD, et al. Lower extremity arteriography with use of iodinated contrast material or gadodiamide to supplement CO_2 angiography in patients with renal insufficiency. J Vasc Interv Radiol 2000;11(1):35–43.

20. Thomsen HS, Almèn T, Morcos SK, et al. Gadolinium-containing contrast media for radiographic examinations: a position paper. Eur Radiol 2002;12(10):2600–5.

21. Ellis JH, Cohan RH, Sonnad SS, et al. Selective use of radiographic low-osmolality contrast media in the 1990s. Radiology 1996;200(2):297–311.

---

[1] {A} = randomized controlled trials and meta-analyses, {B} = other evidence such as well-designed controlled and uncontrolled studies, unlabeled = neither (eg, editorials, literature reviews, case series).

22. McCullough PA, Bertrand ME, Brinker JA, et al. A meta-analysis of the renal safety of isosmolar iodixanol compared with low-osmolar contrast media. J Am Coll Cardiol 2006;48(4):692–9 {A}.

23. Toutant C. GE unit ordered to pay $11.3 million over false-advertising claims against competitor; judge denies competitor's request that GE subsidiary Amersham disgorge $1 billion in profits. Available at: http://www.law.com/jsp/article.jsp?id= 1202429880602. Accessed April 26, 2009.

24. Heinrich MC, Häberle L, Müller V, et al. Nephrotoxicity of iso-osmolar iodixanol compared with nonionic low-osmolar contrast media: meta-analysis of randomized controlled trials. Radiology 2009; 250(1):68–86 {A}.

25. Solomon RJ, Natarajan MK, Doucet S, et al. Cardiac angiography in renally impaired patients (CARE) study: a randomized double-blind trial of contrast-induced nephropathy in patients with chronic kidney disease. Circulation 2007;115:3189–96 {A}.

26. Thomsen HS. Current evidence on prevention and management of contrast-induced nephropathy. Eur Radiol 2007;17(Suppl 6):F33–7.

27. Mueller C, Buerkle G, Buettner HJ, et al. Prevention of contrast media-associated nephropathy: randomized comparison of 2 hydration regimens in 1620 patients undergoing coronary angioplasty. Arch Intern Med 2002;162(3):329–36 {A}.

28. Weisbord SD, Palevsky PM. Prevention of contrast-induced nephropathy with volume expansion. Clin J Am Soc Nephrol 2008;3(1):273–80.

29. Jakobsen JA, Berg KJ, Waaler A, et al. Renal effects of the non-ionic contrast medium iopentol after intravenous injection in healthy volunteers. Acta Radiol 1990;31(1):87–91 {B}.

30. Merten GJ, Burgess WP, Gray LV, et al. Prevention of contrast-induced nephropathy with sodium bicarbonate: a randomized controlled trial. JAMA 2004; 291(19):2328–34 {A}.

31. Adolph E, Holdt-Lehmann B, Chatterjee T, et al. Renal insufficiency following radiocontrast exposure trial (REINFORCE): a randomized comparison of sodium bicarbonate versus sodium chloride hydration for the prevention of contrast-induced nephropathy. Coron Artery Dis 2008;19(6):413–9 {A}.

32. Navaneethan SD, Singh S, Appasamy S, et al. Sodium bicarbonate therapy for prevention of contrast-induced nephropathy: a systematic review and meta-analysis. Am J Kidney Dis 2009;53(4): 617–27 {A}.

33. Ho KM, Morgan DJ. Use of isotonic sodium bicarbonate to prevent radiocontrast nephropathy in patients with mild pre-existing renal impairment: a meta-analysis. Anaesth Intensive Care 2008; 36(5):646–53 {A}.

34. Hogan SE, L'Allier P, Chetcuti S, et al. Current role of sodium bicarbonate-based preprocedural hydration for the prevention of contrast-induced acute kidney injury: a meta-analysis. Am Heart J 2008;156(3): 414–21 {A}.

35. Solomon R, Werner C, Mann D, et al. Effects of saline, mannitol, and furosemide to prevent acute decreases in renal function induced by radiocontrast agents. N Engl J Med 1994;331(21):1416–20 {A}.

36. Dussol B, Morange S, Loundoun A, et al. A randomized trial of saline hydration to prevent contrast nephropathy in chronic renal failure patients. Nephrol Dial Transplant 2006;21(8):2120–6 {A}.

37. Madyoon H, Croushore L, Weaver D, et al. Use of fenoldopam to prevent radiocontrast nephropathy in high-risk patients. Catheter Cardiovasc Interv 2001;53(3):341–5 {B}.

38. Allaqaband S, Tumuluri R, Malik AM, et al. Prospective randomized study of N-acetylcysteine, fenoldopam, and saline for prevention of radiocontrast-induced nephropathy. Catheter Cardiovasc Interv 2002;57(3): 279–83 {A}.

39. Tumlin JA, Wang A, Murray PT, et al. Fenoldopam mesylate blocks reductions in renal plasma flow after radiocontrast dye infusion: a pilot trial in the prevention of contrast nephropathy. Am Heart J 2002;143(5):894–903 {A}.

40. Stone GW, McCullough PA, Tumlin JA, et al. Fenoldopam mesylate for the prevention of contrast-induced nephropathy: a randomized controlled trial. JAMA 2003;290(17):2284–91 {A}.

41. Tepel M, van der Giet M, Schwarzfeld C, et al. Prevention of radiographic-contrast-agent-induced reductions in renal function by acetylcysteine. N Engl J Med 2000;343(3):180–4 {A}.

42. Kelly AM, Dwamena B, Cronin P, et al. Meta-analysis: effectiveness of drugs for preventing contrast-induced nephropathy. Ann Intern Med 2008;148(4): 284–94 {A}.

43. Bagshaw SM, McAlister FA, Manns BJ, et al. Acetylcysteine in the prevention of contrast-induced nephropathy. A case study of the pitfalls in the evolution of evidence. Arch Intern Med 2006; 166(2):161–6.

44. Biondi-Zoccai GGL, Lotrionte M, Abbate A, et al. Compliance with QUOROM and quality of reporting of overlapping meta-analyses on the role of acetylcysteine in the prevention of contrast associated nephropathy: case study. BMJ 2006;332(7535): 202–9.

45. Vaitkus PT, Brar C. N-acetylcysteine in the prevention of contrast-induced nephropathy: publication bias perpetuated by meta-analyses. Am Heart J 2007;153(2):275–80.

46. Van Praet JT, De Vriese AS. Prevention of contrast-induced nephropathy: a critical review. Curr Opin Nephrol Hypertens 2007;16(4):336–47.

47. Hoffmann U, Fischereder M, Krüger B, et al. The value of N-acetylcysteine in the prevention of radio-contrast agent-induced nephropathy seems questionable. J Am Soc Nephrol 2004;15(2):407–10 {B}.

48. Diskin CJ. Creatinine and glomerular filtration rate: evolution of an accommodation. Ann Clin Biochem 2007;44(1):16–9.

49. Preiss DJ, Godber IM, Lamb EJ, et al. The influence of a cooked-meat meal on estimated glomerular filtration rate. Ann Clin Biochem 2007;44(Pt 1):35–42 {B}.

50. Poletti PA, Saudan P, Platon A, et al. IV N-acetyl-cysteine and emergency CT: use of serum creatinine and cystatin C as markers of radiocontrast nephrotoxicity. AJR Am J Roentgenol 2007; 189(3):687–92 {A}.

51. Rehman T, Fought J, Solomon R. N-acetylcysteine effect on serum creatinine and cystatin C levels in CKD patients. Clin J Am Soc Nephrol 2008;3: 1610–4 {B}.

52. Fishbane S, Durhan JH, Marzo K, et al. N-acetylcys-teine in the prevention of radiocontrast-induced nephropathy. J Am Soc Nephrol 2004;15:251–60.

53. Shalansky SJ, Vu T, Pate GE, et al. N-acetylcysteine for prevention of radiographic contrast material-induced nephropathy: is the intravenous route best? Pharmacotherapy 2005;25(8):1095–103.

54. Huber W, Eckel F, Hennig M, et al. Prophylaxis of contrast material-induced nephropathy in patients in intensive care: acetylcysteine, theophylline, or both? A randomized study. Radiology 2006;239(3): 793–804 {B}.

55. Ix JH, McCulloch CE, Chertow GM. Theophylline for the prevention of radiocontrast nephropathy: a meta-analysis. Nephrol Dial Transplant 2004; 19(11):2747–53 {A}.

56. Bagshaw SM, Ghali WA. Theophylline for prevention of contrast-induced nephropathy: a systematic review and meta-analysis. Arch Intern Med 2005; 165(10):1087–93 {A}.

57. Weinstein JM, Heyman S, Brezis M. Potential delete-rious effect of furosemide in radiocontrast nephrop-athy. Nephron 1992;62(4):413–5 {A}.

58. Li G, Yin L, Liu T, et al. Role of probucol in preventing contrast-induced acute kidney injury after coronary interventional procedure. Am J Cardiol 2009; 103(4):512–4 {A}.

59. Boscheri A, Weinbrenner C, Botzek B, et al. Failure of ascorbic acid to prevent contrast-media induced nephropathy in patients with renal dysfunction. Clin Nephrol 2007;68(5):279–86 {A}.

60. Morikawa S, Sone T, Tsuboi H, et al. Renal protective effects and the prevention of contrast-induced nephropathy by atrial natriuretic peptide. J Am Coll Cardiol 2009;53(12):1040–6 {A}.

61. Gupta RK, Kapoor A, Tewari S, et al. Captopril for prevention of contrast-induced nephropathy in dia-betic patients: a randomized study. Indian Heart J 1999;51(5):521–6 {A}.

62. Khoury Z, Schlicht JR, Como J, et al. The effect of prophylactic nifedipine on renal function in patients administered contrast media. Pharmacotherapy 1995;15(1):59–65 {A}.

63. Madsen JK, Jensen W, Sandermann J, et al. Effect of nitrendipine on renal function and on hormonal parameters after intravascular iopromide. Acta Radiol 1998;39(4):375–80 {A}.

64. Sketch MH, Whelton A, Schollmayer E, et al. Preven-tion of contrast media-induced renal dysfunction with prostaglandin E_1: a randomized, double-blind, placebo-controlled. Am J Ther 2001;8(3):155–62 {A}.

65. Koch J-A, Plum J, Grabensee B, et al. Prostaglandin E1: a new agent for the prevention of renal dysfunc-tion in high risk patients caused by radiocontrast media? PGE1 Study Group. Nephrol Dial Transplant 2000;15(1):43–9 {A}.

66. Morcos SK. Prevention of contrast media nephro-toxicity – the story so far. Clin Radiol 2004;59(5): 381–9.

67. Morcos SK. Prevention of contrast media-induced nephrotoxicity after angiographic procedures. J Vasc Interv Radiol 2005;16(1):13–23.

68. Pannu N, Wiebe N, Tonelli M, et al. Prophylaxis strat-egies for contrast-induced nephropathy. JAMA 2006;295(23):2765–79.

69. Stacul F, Adam A, Becker CR, et al. Strategies to reduce the risk of contrast-induced nephropathy. Am J Cardiol 2006;98(Suppl):59k–77k.

70. Thomsen HS, Morcos SK, Barrett BJ. Contrast-induced nephropathy: the wheel has turned 360 degrees. Acta Radiol 2008;49(6):646–57.

71. Sterling KA, Tehrani T, Rudnick MR. Clinical signifi-cance and preventive strategies for contrast induced nephropathy. Curr Opin Nephrol Hypertens 2008;17(6):616–23.

72. Cruz DN, Perazella MA, Bellomo R, et al. Extracor-poreal blood purification therapies for prevention of radiocontrast-induced nephropathy: a systematic review. Am J Kidney Dis 2006;48(3):361–71 {A}.

73. Vogt B, Ferrari P, Schönholzer C, et al. Prophylactic hemodialysis after radiocontrast media in patients with renal insufficiency is potentially harmful. Am J Med 2001;111(9):692–8 {A}.

74. Lehnert T, Keller E, Gondolf K, et al. Effect of haemo-dialysis after contrast medium administration in patients with renal insufficiency. Nephrol Dial Trans-plant 1998;13(2):358–62 {A}.

75. Marenzi G, Lauri G, Campodonico J, et al. Compar-ison of two hemofiltration protocols for prevention of contrast-induced nephropathy in high-risk patients. Am J Med 2005;119(2):155–62 {A}.

76. Marenzi G, Marana I, Lauri G, et al. The prevention of radiocontrast-agent-induced nephropathy by hemofiltration. N Engl J Med 2003;349(14):1333–40 {A}.

77. Elicker BM, Cypel YS, Weinreb JC. IV contrast administration for CT: a survey of practices for the screening and prevention of contrast nephropathy. AJR Am J Roentgenol 2006;186(6):1651–8.

78. Thomsen HS, Morcos SK. Risk of contrast-medium-induced nephropathy in high risk patients undergoing MDCT – a pooled analysis of two randomized trials. Eur Radiol 2009;19(4):891–7 {A}.

79. Barrett BJ, Katzberg RW, Thomsen HS, et al. Contrast-induced nephropathy in patients with chronic kidney disease undergoing computed tomography: a double-blind comparison of iodixanol and iopamidol. Invest Radiol 2006;41(11):815–21 {A}.

80. Thomsen HS, Morcos SK, Erley CM, et al. The ACTIVE Trial: comparison of the effects on renal function of iomeprol-400 and iodixanol-320 in patients with chronic kidney disease undergoing abdominal computed tomography. Invest Radiol 2008;43(3):170–8 {A}.

81. Katzberg RW, Barrett BJ. Risk of iodinated contrast material-induced nephropathy with intravenous administration. Radiology 2007;243(3):622–8.

82. Morcos SK, Thomsen HS, Webb JA, et al. Dialysis and contrast media. Eur Radiol 2002;12(12):3026–30.

Carbon Dioxide in Angiography to Reduce the Risk of Contrast-Induced Nephropathy

Irvin F. Hawkins, MD[a],*, Kyung J. Cho, MD, FACR[b],
James G. Caridi, MD[a]

KEYWORDS

• Digital subtraction angiography • Carbon dioxide
• Plastic bag delivery system • Arteries • Stents
• Angioplasty • Embolization • Veins

Carbon dioxide (CO_2) is a nontoxic, invisible gas that is highly compressible, nonviscous, buoyant, and rapidly absorbed. It is 20 times more soluble than oxygen. CO_2 is not only rapidly dissolved in the blood but, when delivered intravenously, is eliminated by one pass through the lungs. Most importantly, CO_2, as an intravascular imaging agent, lacks both allergic potential and renal toxicity. Moreover, its low viscosity (1/400 that of iodinated contrast) provides unique qualities useful in both angiographic diagnosis and intervention.

Currently, CO_2 has been used as an intravascular alternative to iodinated contrast material for over three decades. Although it is dissimilar to routine contrast and requires a unique delivery system, it has been routinely used successfully as an adjunct to liquid contrast in patients in renal failure and those allergic to contrast. It is not the quintessential contrast agent and often requires more meticulous manipulation to produce the desired images. In the past, fool-proof, safe delivery of CO_2 was very difficult. However, a converted fluid management plastic bag delivery system has now been used for the last 14 years, and is both faster and easier than injecting iodinated contrast. More importantly, the delivery system is almost completely fail-safe.[1]

With the advent of MR angiography and CT angiography, the diagnostic use of CO_2 digital subtraction angiography (DSA) has declined significantly. Recently, however, there has been resurgence because of gadolinium-induced nephrogenic systemic fibrosis (NSF) in patients with advanced reduction in renal function.[2] Therefore, if an angiographic examination is necessary in patients with renal impairment, the choices may potentiate either NSF from the gadolinium- or contrast-induced nephropathy from iodinated contrast. Alternatively, CO_2 DSA can be used safely in many of these cases. Additionally, intravascular CO_2 use has also increased because of the recent discoveries of more useful applications, as well as the increasing complexity of cases requiring greater contrast doses. CO_2 can be used in unlimited doses without jeopardizing the kidney.

UNIQUE PROPERTIES OF CO_2

CO_2 is invisible, buoyant, compressible, and nonviscous. These unique properties can provide

[a] Department of Radiology, University of Florida College of Medicine, 1600 SW Archer Road, Box 100374, Gainesville, FL 32610, USA
[b] Department of Radiology, University of Michigan Medical Center, 1500 East Medical Center Drive, Ann Arbor, MI 48109-0030, USA
* Corresponding author.
E-mail address: hawkii@radiology.ufl.edu (I.F. Hawkins).

Radiol Clin N Am 47 (2009) 813–825
doi:10.1016/j.rcl.2009.07.002
0033-8389/09/$ – see front matter © 2009 Published by Elsevier Inc.

distinct advantages and disadvantages in angiographic procedures. As an endogenous gas, it is nonallergic, nonnephrotoxic, and its viscosity is 1/400 that of iodinated contrast and, therefore, can disseminate more readily than liquid contrast. Because it is a gas, CO_2 is invisible, and air contamination must be avoided. Moreover, even without contamination, administration of the gas into the cerebral vessels is an absolute contraindication.

As opposed to liquid contrast, CO_2 does not mix with blood. It is buoyant and will rise to the nondependent portion of a large diameter vessel. Therefore, to assure accurate representation of a vascular structure the entirety of blood in the imaged vessel should be displaced. Incomplete displacement can lead to spurious imaging (i.e. smaller vessels or larger percentage stenoses).

Because CO_2 is compressible, steps must be taken to avoid excessive volumes and explosive delivery. If compressed, a 20-cc syringe can hold 200 ccs of CO_2. This exposes the patient to possible excessive and explosive delivery, which can lead to undesired reflux and rapid expansion of vessels, which could cause untoward symptoms, such as pain, nausea, and vomiting following CO_2 injection into the abdominal aorta, celiac, or superior mesenteric artery. Advantages and disadvantages of CO_2 are presented in **Box 1**.

WHY SHOULD I LEARN HOW TO USE CO_2?

Presently, with advances in delivery and imaging systems, CO_2 can be safely used in patients at risk for adverse reactions to iodine- or gadolinium-based contrast agents for most diagnostic and interventional procedures. In addition, CO_2 has definite advantages for many interventional procedures. The authors' 38-year experience in over 6,000 patients and review of the literature have shown that CO_2 is the only safe angiographic contrast for patients with a history of serious allergic reactions to iodinated contrast media and in patients with renal failure. Contrast-induced nephropathy (CIN) and NSF are serious complications that should be avoided. As discussed in detail elsewhere in this issue of *The Clinics*, these complications are associated with marked increase in morbidity and mortality of the affected patients.

LACK OF RENAL TOXICITY OF CO_2

Animal studies in canines showed that selective CO_2 injection in renal arteries had no significant effect on renal function or histology, with the exception of one dog that sustained a minimal

---

Box 1
Advantage and disadvantages of CO_2

Advantages

Nonallergic

Nonneprhotoxic

Low viscosity—easily delivered via microcatheter, between catheter and guidewire, flows readily into bleeding sites and from paremchymal injections into the venous system

Can inject larger volumes via small catheter with reflux resulting in CO_2 filling of proximal vessels

Cost

Disadvantages

Invisible, allowing potential for undetected contamination

Requires a unique delivery system

Gas is compressible

Contraindicated in the cerebral and coronary circulation and thoracic aorta

Bowel gas and motion can reduce or eliminate image quality

Obtaining quality diagnostic images may be more labor intense

---

degree of acute tubular necrosis. This animal endured multiple selective renal CO_2 injections while the dog's kidney was positioned above the injection catheter, resulting in trapped CO_2 and minimal ischemia.[3] A more recent study in rats[4] comparing renal cortical and medullary blood flow with CO_2 versus ioxaglate showed that the marked decrease in medullary flow with ioxaglate was absent with CO_2.

As far as the authors are aware, there are no reports in the published literature of CO_2 causing CIN. The authors' clinical experience in using CO_2 for angiography in patients with renal failure and renal transplant patients (over 100 patients)[5] has been extremely encouraging, with no technical complications or important deterioration in renal function. In renal transplant patients, CO_2 angiography is more effective because of the anterior position of the transplanted kidney, which allows good filling of the renal arteries with CO_2, much better than in the native kidney, which has a posterior-oriented position.

The right renal artery always fills with aortic injections; however, the more posterior located left renal artery occasionally is difficult to image. Using the plastic bag system injecting smaller volumes (30 cc) of CO_2 with nonexplosive delivery and an end-hole catheter, the left renal artery is much more frequently seen (Fig. 1). If, after one or two abdominal injections, the left renal artery is not seen, the authors either selectively catheterize this artery or elevate the left side of the patient. If these maneuvers are not successful, placing the patient in the right lateral decubitus position always results in filling the left renal artery with CO_2 if it is patent.

IMPORTANT FEATURES OF CO_2
Low Viscosity

The low viscosity of CO_2 increases its sensitivity in detecting acute hemorrhage, arteriovenous shunting, collateral vessels, and arteriovenous shunting in tumors. The low viscosity also allows easy administration of CO_2 into microcatheters and permits injection between the catheter and guidewire, eliminating the need to remove the guidewire from the target organ after intervention. This makes CO_2 an ideal contrast agent for interventional procedures, such as angioplasty and stent placement and verifying the exact position of the needle or catheter before a larger catheter or device is placed in a potentially dangerous location. With wedged hepatic and splenic arterial injection and injection into the hepatic parenchyma and splenic pulp, the low viscosity facilitates visualization of the portal veins without causing histologic damage.

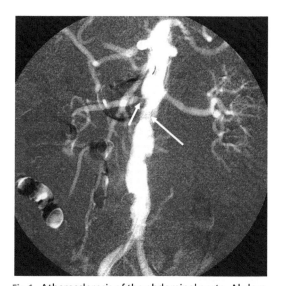

Fig.1. Atherosclerosis of the abdominal aorta. Abdominal aortogram (DSA technique) with 30 cc of CO_2 shows markedly irregular wall and narrowing (*long arrow*) of the infrarenal aorta. There is a severe stenosis at origin of the right renal artery (*short arrow*). The left renal artery is patent, with good distal perfusion.

Reflux

The gaseous property of CO_2 results in central reflux from the point of administration. This permits central assessment of the feeding vessels without the need for catheter withdrawal to improve central visualization that might be required with iodinated contrast agents. This is exemplified by the placement of renal stents and the need to identify the appropriate position of the ostium and stenosis. Using CO_2 injection through the sheath with the stent-mounted balloon catheter in place, and between the balloon catheter and guide wire, the location of the more central stenosis can be assessed and the stent positioned with precision.

POTENTIAL COMPLICATIONS OF CO_2
Excessive Volumes

Injecting excessive volumes of CO_2 is probably one of the most serious potential complications and might lead to drop in blood pressure, bradycardia, and elevation of the ST segments in EKG. The authors experienced this complication only once with one patient after inadvertently injecting over 3,000 cc of CO_2 during a transjugular intrahepatic portosystemic shunt (TIPS) procedure. The patient was placed in the left lateral decubitus position with immediate normalization of vital signs and EKG. With the right side elevated, the buoyant gas shifted to the higher right atrium and the blood flew under the gas to perfuse the pulmonary artery. The patient's survival can be attributed to the extreme solubility of CO_2. In another patient, after injection over 2,000 cc of CO_2 into an abdominal aortic aneurysm (AAA), the patient developed severe diarrhea, with follow-up endoscopy demonstrating colonic ischemia. The trapped CO_2 prevented flow into the inferior mesenteric artery (IMA) for over 1 hour and the gas, which does not mix with blood, produced a barrier preventing normal collateral blood flow. Fortunately, the colon was found to be normal 2 weeks later during the AAA surgery.

More recently, the authors have performed an extensive venous study in 20 swine,[6] injecting the equivalent of 50 cc to 600 cc of CO_2 in man. There were no untoward events and little or no changes in blood gases, pH, or pulmonary or arterial blood pressure when the equivalent of 100 cc was injected. However, when an amount comparable to 600 cc was injected, there was one death. It was noted that as the volume of CO_2 was increased, the pulmonary pressure increased incrementally. Although the authors have not experienced any cerebral complications, theoretically, if the pulmonary pressure increases markedly, a potentially patent foramen ovale may open and the CO_2 could flow into the left atrium and subsequently into the aortic arch.

To prevent any possibility of injecting excessive volumes of CO_2, the patient should never be connected directly to the CO_2 cylinder. The cylinder typically contains over 3 million cc of compressed gas at very high pressure. If a stopcock is turned in the wrong direction, the cylinder can unload directly into the vascular system. Even a syringe connected directly to a cylinder can contain an excessive volume. Because of Boyle's law, the volume of CO_2 decreases with increased pressure. If the cylinder's CO_2 regulator is set at a high psi, a hand syringe will be filled with a higher volume of CO_2. If a finite-volume plastic bag delivery system is used, there is no possibility of injecting excessive or inaccurate volumes. When the CO_2 source (plastic bag) is at atmospheric pressure (flaccid plastic bag), whatever volume is aspirated from the source will be the exact volume in the syringe.

AIR CONTAMINATION

An uncompromised closed-delivery system is crucially important to avoid air contamination. Cho and colleagues[7] have shown that if the stopcock of a syringe remains open, the extremely diffusible CO_2 in the syringe is quickly replaced with room air, regardless of the syringe's position. The differential in partial pressure between CO_2 in the syringe and in the room air causes room air to diffuse into the syringe with the open stopcock at a rate of 0.2 cc per second, with air replacing the majority of the CO_2 within 20 minutes. Thus, it is very important to use a leak-proof closed system to prevent potential lethal air complications.

Indications of CO_2 Angiography

CO_2 is used primarily for angiography, with the exception of the cerebral or coronary circulations in patients with iodinated contrast allergy and renal failure. It permits multiple, safe injections for renal transplant evaluation and intervention. CO_2 is also very beneficial in complex interventional procedures, where it can be used alone or in combination with iodinated contrast to minimize the risk of renal complications and volume-overload problems in patients with congestive heart failure. Because of the rapid dissolution and one-pass elimination by the lungs, there is no maximum CO_2 dose when less than 100 cc is injected every 2 minutes. In addition, using the closed plastic bag delivery system, CO_2 can be very expediently injected as a contrast agent in any luminal structure, such as the biliary tree, urinary tract, abscess cavity, and fistula.

The very low-viscosity of CO_2 can occasionally provide additional information, otherwise not obtainable with iodinated contrast. In addition to the previously mentioned advantages of the low viscosity of CO_2, the authors have noted that when CO_2 was used during embolization the tumors have appeared totally ablated with liquid contrast but were only partially embolized, as noted with subsequent CO_2 injections. Because embolization procedures alone can exacerbate renal failure and many are high risk,[8] the authors are routinely using the many unique properties of CO_2 for most oncologic procedures. For TIPS procedures (**Fig. 2**),[9] evaluation of portal

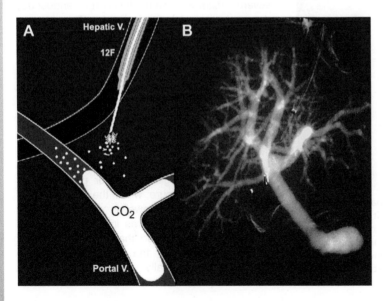

Fig. 2. CO_2 prenchymal hepatic injection with fine needle for TIPS. (*A*) Diagram of portal vein targeting: 21-gauge needle advanced 1 cm through hepatic vein into parenchyma, injecting 30 cc of CO_2 forcefully. (*B*) Entire portal system filled, including extra hepatic portal vein.

hypertension and occlusion, and portal vein embolization, the low-viscosity also permits filling of the portal system much more reliably than iodinated contrast, either by wedged hepatic vein injections, direct injections into the parenchyma of the liver, or via a fine-needle in the splenic pulp[10] and injection into peripheral hepatic arteries. CO_2 passes very easily through the sinusoids into the portal system against the direction of blood flow. CO_2 is also ideal for the filling of central veins from distal injection sites (25-gauge needle in hand vein) and frequently, in patients with venous thrombosis, it is the only contrast that will opacify the more central system, permitting accurate assessment and successful intervention (Fig. 3). It can be used effectively for inferior vena cava (IVC) filter placement, even at the bedside.[11] There is a recent report of CO_2 use for intraosseous venography in percutaneous vertebroplasty.[12]

Recently, CO_2 has been used in high-risk endovascular aneurysm repair procedures to reduce CIN and has been effective in demonstrating endoleaks.[13–15] This was underscored in a case where a covered stent was placed to repair a lacerated superficial femoral artery (Fig. 4). The leak was detected only after CO_2 was employed.

ABSOLUTE CONTRAINDICATIONS

Studies of CO_2 carotid injections in rats, dogs, and rabbits[16,17] have suggested that CO_2 could be neurotoxic. Because of possible neurotoxicity and cardiac ischemia,[18] the cerebral and coronary arterial circulation should never be exposed to CO_2. The authors never inject CO_2 in the prone position because the buoyancy will fill spinal arteries and may cause spinal cord ischemia. Never administer CO_2 with the patient's head in an elevated position because the buoyant CO_2 can flow countercurrent and cause possible reflux into the cerebral circulation. Because of the possibility of central reflux into the cerebral circulation, CO_2 should not be used to evaluate the arterial

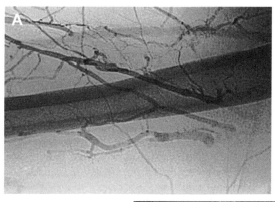
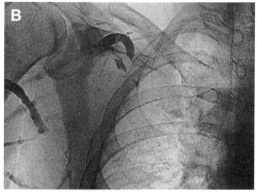
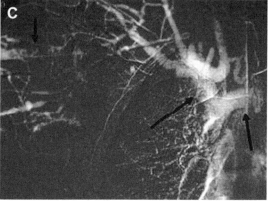

Fig. 3. Right axillosubclavian vein thrombosis in a 31-year-old man with right arm swelling and recent pulmonary embolism. (A) Right arm venogram with iodinated contrast shows no filling of the brachial or axillary veins secondary to thrombosis. (B) Only a few isolated veins are filled in the shoulder and axilla. (C) CO_2 venogram again shows occlusion of the axillary and subsubclavian veins with acute thrombus in cephalic vein (shorter arrow). There is excellent filling of the right and left innominate veins (long arrows) and the superior vena cava (SVC) secondary to the low viscosity of CO_2, which guided a successful catheter-directed fibrinolysis.

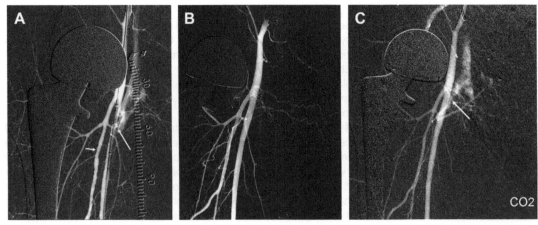

Fig. 4. Endoleak seen only with CO_2 in a patient with a lacerated femoral artery. (*A*) Injection of 10 cc of CO_2 as the covered stent catheter was positioned at the bleeding site of a superficial femoral artery laceration with shunting into the femoral vein (*longer arrow*). After the stent was deployed, the hemorrhage stopped. Note the irregular wall along the deep femoral artery (*shorter arrow*) representing stationary arterial wave. (*B*) One day after stent placement, the patient clinically was massively bleeding; however, injection of 20 cc of iodinated contrast showed no evidence of extravasation. (*C*) Injection of 10 cc of CO_2 immediately after the iodinated injection showed type one endoleak (*arrow*), which was treated successfully by over-dilating the stent graft.

limb of dialysis fistula. It can, however, be used cautiously for evaluating the venous limb.

RELATIVE CONTRAINDICATIONS

The authors do not use CO_2 in conjunction with nitrous oxide anesthesia during CO_2 studies, because in animals it has been found that partial pressure differentials of the nitrous oxide saturated in the soft tissues will diffuse into the CO_2 bubble, increasing its volume by approximately six times. The CO_2 bubble may increase from 100 cc of injected CO_2 to 600 cc, which in the venous system may cause significant problems (vapor lock of the pulmonary artery). If only small volumes of CO_2 are required, nitrous oxide could be used safely if there is no alternative contrast available.

The authors have used CO_2 in hundreds of patients with pulmonary compromise without complications; however, the volumes are reduced and a greater delay between injections allows more time for the CO_2 to be absorbed.

In patients who present with intestinal ischemia or an AAA, the authors reduce the number of injections and volumes and allow more time between injections, permitting absorption of the CO_2. If the gas remains trapped in the aneurysm, the patient's position is changed to free the gas.

CO_2 DELIVERY

The delivery of CO_2 has evolved over the past 38 years. It has included many different manual delivery systems, with or without manifolds, as well as more than five dedicated automated controlled systems. Many of these were not user friendly and never approved by the Food and Drug Administration. Previously, during bench testing of these devices, the authors discovered multiple potential complications but experienced a few clinical complications, which were short-lived.

After more than 20 years of experimenting with many different systems, the authors introduced a plastic bag system, as well as a technique of delivery extrapolated from their experience with computer-controlled injectors. The plastic bag system has proven to be very user friendly and actually much faster and easier than liquid angiographic injectors or hand delivery systems. If assembled correctly, its only disadvantage is the ease of making rapid injections in regions where ischemia could occur if injections are made more frequently, without time for the CO_2 to reabsorb.

Because the plastic bag, which only contains 1,500 cc at atmospheric pressure (if it is not distended), there is no possibility of inadvertently injecting excessive volumes and virtually no probability of air contamination if one uses the system properly. The authors have used this system for over 12 years without complications. In the last 8 years, improvements have been instituted that further reduce the probability of air contamination (**Fig. 5**).[1]

The authors feel that it is extremely important to employ a disposable aluminum cylinder containing United States Pharmacopeia (USP) grade

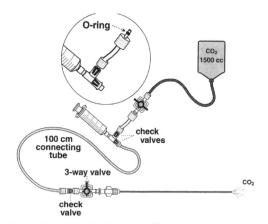

Fig. 5. Current plastic bag delivery system showing details of the O-ring gas fitting, which prevents air aspiration during delivery syringe filling. The one-way check valves eliminate stopcock manipulation and prevent back bleeding into the angiographic catheter. The distal three-way stopcock is used to clear the air from the distal fittings and inject drugs or iodinated contrast, keeping the system closed at all times. The authors now flush the catheter every 3 to 5 minutes with CO_2 instead of saline.

(99.99%) CO_2 with high purity gas fittings and regulators. The cylinder is supplied with a special spring-loaded push-button valve. These disposable cylinders are individually checked for CO_2 purity. The authors also use a 0.2-micron filter to eliminate any particulate or microbial contaminates. This filter is attached to the spring-loaded push-button valve. The bag will only fill when the button is depressed. If a cylinder is used without this spring valve, which closes automatically, the cylinder may empty in a few hours if the main valve is inadvertently left partially open.

The present system is very user-friendly, requiring less than 3 minutes to fill and flush the CO_2 bag. The bag is filled and emptied three times via a short sterile connecting tube and a standard three-way valve connected to the submicron filter. Sterility is maintained by keeping the bag on the angiographic table to be sure the delivery component is securely connected to the plastic bag. It is recommended to initially overfill the bag one time, manually squeezing to check for a gas leaks. The bag is connected to the delivery system, which has an O-ring gas fitting and multiple one-way check flow valves, which obviate stopcock manipulation. The distal check valve inhibits blood from filling the angiographic catheter. Repeated injections can be made very rapidly simply by aspirating and injecting. All the connections are glued by the manufacture with a 100-cm connecting tube between the delivery syringe and the distal high-pressure three-way stopcock. The extension

tube permits the operator to stand behind a protective radiation barrier during the injections. The distal high-pressure three-way stopcock, which is connected to the angiographic catheter, is used to remove air from the stopcock by back-bleeding the angiographic catheter and then closing the stopcock to the patient and flushing the stopcock with CO_2 three times, resulting in a pure CO_2-blood interface. After a forceful injection of 5 cc of CO_2 is made to clear the blood from the catheter, the system is ready for multiple nonexplosive CO_2 injections and imaging. The high-pressure three-way stopcock can also be used to administer drugs or inject iodinated contrast, either by hand or angiographic injector. It can also be used to discharge excess CO_2 from the delivery syringe, maintaining a closed system without chance of air contamination at all times. The distal three-way stopcock is never used for CO_2 delivery because if the port closest to the plastic bag is open, air will be aspirated as the syringe is filled. This is the only way air can be inadvertently injected.

The system can also be used for interventional procedures if a specialized side-arm O-ring fitting is attached. This permits injection of the low-viscosity CO_2 between the guidewire and the catheter, or guidewire and any size needle. Injection of relatively large amounts of CO_2 between the guidewire and catheter permits accurate visualization of vascular anatomy before, during, and after interventional procedures (balloon dilatation, stent placement, or placement of larger potentially dangerous catheters, and so forth). A large syringe and considerable force is required to purge the liquid from the small space between the catheter and the guidewire or needle. There is a prolonged delay of many seconds; however, when the liquid is cleared, the syringe's plunger moves forward easily and subsequent injections can be made rapidly with little effort.

Hospital stores can provide a CO_2 cylinder that is filled with pure USP grade gas; however, frequently the tanks are cast iron and may contain rust and other contaminates. Again, the authors strongly suggest obtaining a disposable cylinder, with gas-type fittings, that has been individually tested for purity. When a new cylinder is delivered, 15 cc to 20 cc of CO_2 should be injected into the venous system imaging the pulmonary artery, to be absolutely sure that there is no air contamination. The CO_2 will trap in the anterior-located main pulmonary artery and will absorb within 15 to 20 seconds. It is easily seen with routine fluoroscopy; however, the pulmonary artery can be more accurately visualized with DSA (Fig. 6). If it remains longer, there is a possibility of air contamination.

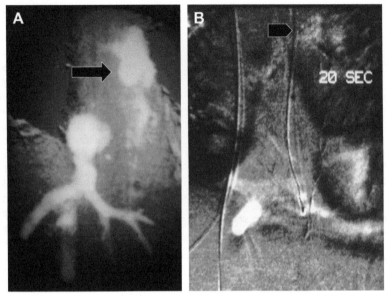

Fig. 6. Method to detect possible air contamination of CO_2. (A) For TIPS procedure or any venous study when multiple injections are anticipated, a hepatic vein or any vein is injected imaging the pulmonary artery. Initially CO_2 traps in most anterior main pulmonary artery (arrow). (B) After 15 to 20 seconds, the majority of CO_2 will dissolve because of extreme solubility of CO_2 in blood (arrowhead). If CO_2 remains longer than 20 seconds, one should suspect air contamination.

A closed system without any possibility of valves connecting to the exterior is absolutely necessary to prevent air contamination. With the present plastic bag system, it is extremely important to connect the bag to the delivery system properly. A 30 cc to 60 cc Luer-lock delivery syringe is connected to the end where the O-ring gas fitting is attached. A label stating delivery port is attached. After the plastic bag is filled, the delivery system is also flushed three times. Do not add stopcocks and never connect the delivery system to the CO_2 cylinder. There is never a need to refill the plastic bag (1,500 cc is always more than enough). To be sure there are no leaks in the delivery connections, the one-way bag's stopcock is closed and the delivery syringe is forcefully aspirated. If there is a leak in the tubing or the fittings, the syringe will fill with room air. If the system is sealed, the operator is able to only retract the syringe's plunger a short distance.

During the last 12 years the authors have not flushed the catheter with saline because CO_2 plus water produces carbonic acid and discomfort. The catheter is flushed every 2 to 5 minutes with CO_2.

General principles for CO_2 delivery are as follows:

Be absolutely sure that you are using a pure source of CO_2 USP (99.9%). CO_2 may be used to fill the cylinder; however, the cylinder itself may be contaminated with rust, bacteria, methane or some other contaminate. It is recommended to use a disposable cylinder individually tested for purity.

Use a delivery system where there is no possibility of injecting excessive volumes of CO_2. The flaccid plastic bag prevents inaccurate and inadvertent injections of excessive volumes.

Use a closed system to prevent air contamination. The CO_2 cylinder, which contains over 3,000,000 cc, should never be connected to the closed system. Always maintain the closed integrity of the system. Never use additional stopcocks. When using the plastic bag delivery system, be sure that all ports are closed and that the delivery syringe is attached adjacent to the gas-fitting port for the plastic bag.

Prevent explosive delivery. Purging liquid (blood or saline) from the angiographic catheter prior to CO_2 delivery results in a more consistent delivery, with less discomfort and less breakup into small bubbles.

Initially inject small volumes of CO_2 (30 cc for aortograpy and 5 cc to 10 cc for most selective injections) and increase or decrease the injection rate and volume depending upon the vascular bed that is being imaged.

Wait 2 minutes between injections, depending upon the volume injected and ischemic tolerance of the vascular bed. In high-risk areas, such as abdominal aneurysms, intestinal ischemia, or severe pulmonary compromise, the authors suggest waiting approximately 5 minutes between injections.

In poor flow conditions, elevate the area of interest (legs 10° to 15°, renal arteries 30° to 45°), and if the renal arteries cannot be filled, use the cross-table decubitus position. Alternatively, placing the catheter's tip close to the area of interest will also improve filling.

Injecting vasodilators (nitroglycerin 100 mcg to 150 mcg) intra-arterially into the vascular bed prior to CO_2 delivery improves filling considerably.

Any type radio-opaque-tipped catheter can be used; however, a single end-hole catheter causes less breakup into small bubbles.

DSA imaging: Use a 1,024 × 1,024 high-resolution system with a high-framing rate (4–6 frames per second). Most equipment manufacturers provide a software package that increases photon flux to improve visualization of this low-negative contrast agent, and a stacking program, which integrates multiple frames to produce a single diagnostic composite image.

If the operator has not used the delivery system previously, the following recommendations are suggested:

Assemble the bag and delivery system and practice injecting the CO_2 via a catheter into a container filled with water. Inject both with the angiographic catheter and, for interventional procedures between the guidewire and the catheter, between the needle and a guidewire using a specialized side-arm O-ring fitting.

The integrity of the connection to the bag should be tested frequently by closing the stopcock to the plastic bag and forcefully aspirating.

After one feels comfortable with the system's setup and the delivery technique, the DSA imaging should be tested with the injection of 20 cc of CO_2 into an iliac or a peripheral vein. If the images demonstrate poor contrast (gray), the angiographic equipment applications person should be contacted to change the acquisition parameters. Do not perform your first procedure when iodinated contrast cannot be used.

Furthermore, to ensure the purity of every new CO_2 cylinder, the authors suggest making a venous injection (SVC, IVC, right atrium, or even a peripheral vein) and imaging the pulmonary artery to see if the trapped CO_2 disappears from the pulmonary artery within 15 to 20 seconds. If it remains longer, air contamination is a possibility. Injection of 20 cc of room air is not lethal; however, multiple large volume injections may be disastrous.

Current procedural parameters are as follows:

Runoff (pelvis and lower extremity)
a. Initially, obtain both leg runoffs with the catheter in the distal aorta.
b. Inject 20 cc to 40 cc in 1 second.
c. Elevate the feet 10° to 15° for optimal filling and obtain images of pelvis, thigh, knee, lower legs, and feet.
d. If the IMA is filled and the patient experiences pain, urge to defecate, or has symptoms of intestinal ischemia, the injections should be aborted or the injections should be made more distally in either femoral artery, where the IMA will not be filled.
e. If there is no stacking program, a longer injection (approximately 60 cc over 2 to 3 seconds) is necessary.

Single leg runoff with selective common iliac or more distal femoral arterial injections produce better filling and are unlikely to cause intestinal ischemia. This is the authors' presently preferred method.
a. Perform a selective (antegrade is preferable) injection of the common femoral or more distal arteries. Positioning can be either "over-the-hill" or antegrade placement of a 4 French catheter in the contralateral extremity. If distal filling is suboptimal, a microcatheter can be passed through the antegrade catheter and advanced as distally as possible (Fig. 7). For ipsilateral vessels, retract the catheter to the distal external iliac artery.
b. With stacking, inject 20 cc in 2 seconds. If filling remains poor, inject 20 cc to 40 cc over 3 to 4 seconds.
c. Without stacking, begin with 20 cc to 40 cc over 3 to 4 seconds.
d. Intra-arterial nitroglycerine, 100 mcg to 150 mcg prior to injection.

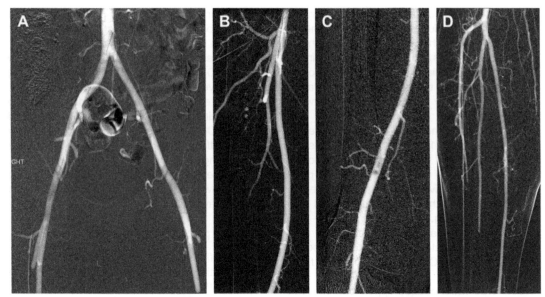

Fig. 7. Coaxial catheterization for preoperative lower extremity arteriogram in a 48-year-old man with ameloblastom of the mandible. (A) Normal CO_2 pelvic arteriogram using an end-hoe catheter (shepherd's hook catheter). (B) Right superficial femoral arteriogram was performed with the shepherd's hook catheter positioned in the proximal superficial femoral artery. (C) The 3-French microcatheter was passed coaxially for the popliteal arteriogram. The popliteal artery is normal. (D) The popliteal artery and its trifurcation branches are normal. Both tibial and peroneal arteries are patent. The volume of CO_2 injected, ranged from 20 cc to 30 cc every 2 seconds.

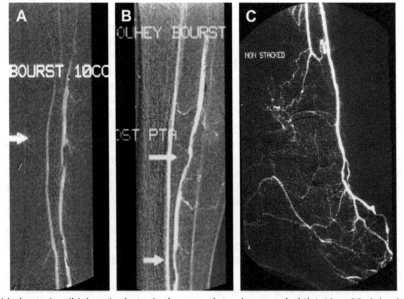

Fig. 8. CO_2-guided anterior tibial angioplasty via the contralateral approach. (A) A 10-cc CO_2 injection via a 300-cm coronary angioplasty catheter demonstrates a 99% stenosis (arrow) of the mid-anterior tibial artery and 50% stenosis of its lower one-third. (B) With a specialized side-arm O-ring fitting multiple CO_2 injections were made with the 0.018-inch guidewire positioned distal to the lesions. Postangioplasty image shows only very minimal residual stenosis (arrows). (C) Good filling of the foot and of dorsalis pedis artery and other unnamed collaterals, again injecting between the guidewire and the balloon catheter. No vasodilators or stacking was required. If iodinated contrast were used, very large amounts of contrast for each injection would have been required via a large guiding catheter at the aortic bifurcation.

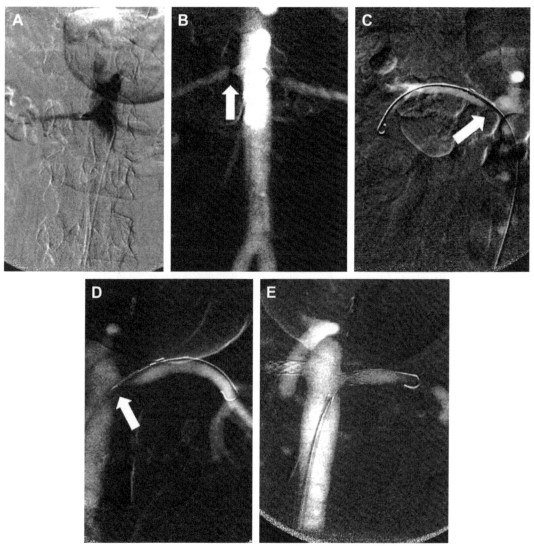

Fig. 9. Bilateral renal stent placement. (*A*) Selective iodinated contrast injection of the right renal artery shows a tight stenosis without any filling of the distal renal arteries. (*B*) A similar injection of 20 cc of CO_2 shows the tight stenosis (*arrow*) plus more distal filling of the right renal artery and a 50% stenosis of the origin of the left renal artery. (*C*) Injection between the stent catheter and the Rosen wire with reflux into the aorta demonstrates that the stent has advanced too distally (*arrow*). (*D*) Injection between the Rosen wire and the stent catheter demonstrating that the stent has been advanced several millimeters too distally into the left renal artery (*arrow*). (*E*) Final CO_2 injection between the guiding catheter and the Rosen wire showing excellent position and patency of both stents.

Aortogram

a. Twenty years ago, the authors injected 200 cc in 2 seconds with a computer-controlled injector, with occasional nausea, abdominal discomfort, urge to defecate, and more nausea when glucagon was used.

b. During the last 14 years, with the nonexplosive plastic bag system the authors have reduced the volume to 30 cc in half a second with less nausea, and if bowel gas obscures the image glucagon may be used.

c. The left renal artery is more difficult to image and may be better visualized by elevating that side. If necessary, a selective injection with a shepherd hook catheter (10 cc–20 cc CO_2 in 1 second) can be performed. Do not inject with patient in the prone position because the lumbar arteries will always fill with potential unknown neurotoxic effects.

d. Selective injections of the visceral arteries commonly require 5 cc to 30 cc in 1 to 2 seconds.

Venous: always image the pulmonary artery after the first injection to rule out air contamination (persistent gas). Normally, CO_2 should disappear after 10 to 20 seconds.

a. SVC and IVC: 20 cc to 50 cc in 1 to 2 seconds.
b. Subclavian: 20 cc to 40 cc in 1 to 2 seconds.
c. Peripheral veins: 15 cc to 25 cc in 4 to 8 seconds, usually with 22-gauge Angio-catheter. Rapid injection precipitates pain.

Interventional procedures
a. Using a specialized side-arm O-ring fitting, CO_2 can be injected between the guide-wire and needle or catheter
b. Use a 20 cc to 50 cc Luer-locked syringe. With a smaller syringe, CO_2 will simply compress without injecting.
c. Wait 5 to 10 seconds for CO_2 to exit the catheter. CO_2 will compress as it purges fluid from the catheter.
d. After purging, subsequent injections require less pressure and delay.

For angioplasty, stent placement, and fibroly-sis (renal, superior mesenteric artery, iliac) over the aortic bifurcation with distal inter-vention (Fig. 8), CO_2 can be injected between the guidewire and the stent cath-eter to verify its exact position before the stent is deployed. For renal stent place-ment, the extreme buoyancy of the gas always results in reflux into the aorta, which visualizes the exact positions of the renal artery ostium (Fig. 9).

TIPS: Using any needle, inject 30 cc of CO_2 into the hepatic parenchyma for visualiza-tion of the portal vein throughout the various steps of the procedure. With the guidewire in place, CO_2 can be injected between the needle and the guidewire to verify the needle entry site and determine stent positioning.

SUMMARY

Clinical experience with the use of CO_2 as a contrast agent has shown that it is safe, and in patients with renal impairment can prevent CIN and the associated morbidity and mortality of this complication. In addition, CO_2 contrast-enhanced examinations may offer more diagnostic information than standard techniques with iodine-based contrast agents in several clinical applica-tions. Equipment advances and competence in using CO_2 delivery systems made imaging with CO_2 a reliable technique for diagnostic and inter-ventional procedures. Utilization of both CO_2 and liquid contrast also increases the safety and effi-cacy of many procedures.

REFERENCES

1. Hawkins IF, Caridi J, Klioze S, et al. Modified plastic bag system with O-ring fitting connection for carbon dioxide angiography. Am J Roentgenol 2001;176(1):229–32.
2. Deo A, Fogel M, Cowper S. Nephrgenic systemic fibrosis: a population study examining the relation-ship of disease development to gadolinium expo-sure. Clin J Am Soc Nephrol 2007;2:264–7.
3. Hawkins IF Jr, Mladinich CR, Storm B, et al. Short-term effects of selective renal arterial carbon dioxide administration on the dog kidney. J Vasc Interv Radiol 1994;5:149–54.
4. Palm F, Bergqvist D, Carlisson PO, et al. The effects of carbon dioxide versus ioxaglate in the rat kidney. J Vasc Interv Radiol 2005;16:269–74.
5. Hawkins IF. Digital subtraction angiography for renal transplants. In: Cho KJ, Hawkins IF, editors. Carbon dioxide angiography: principles, techniques and practices. New York: Informa Healthcare; 2007. p. 104–6.
6. Cho KJ. CO_2 as a venous contrast agent: safety and tolerance. In: Cho KJ, Hawkins IF, editors. Carbon dioxide angiography: principles, techniques and practices. New York: Informa Healthcare; 2007. p. 37–44.
7. Cho DR, Cho KJ, Hawkins IF. Potential air contami-nation during CO_2 angiography using a hand–held syringe: theoretical considerations and gas chroma-tography. Cardiovasc Intervent Radiol 2006;29: 637–41.
8. Huo TI, Wu JC, Kee PC, et al. Incidence and risk factors for acute renal failure in patients with HCC undergoing TACE: a prospective study. Liver Int 2004;24:210–5.
9. Hawkins IF Jr, Johnson AW, Caridi JG, et al. CO_2 fine-needle TIPS. J Vasc Interv Radiol 1997;8:235–9.
10. Caridi J, Hawkins I, Cho K, et al. CO_2 splenoportog-raphy: preliminary results. Am J Roentgenol 2003; 180:1375–8.
11. Sing RF, Stackhouse DJ, Jacobs DJ, et al. Safety and accuracy of bedside carbon dioxide cavogra-phy for insertion of inferior vena cava filters in the intensive care unit. J Am Coll Surg 2001;192(2): 168–71.
12. Tanigawa N, Komenushi A, Kariya S, et al. Intraoss-eous venography with carbon dioxide contrast agent in percutaneous.vertebroplasty. Am J Roent-genol 2005;184:567–70.

13. Kessel DO, Robertson I, Patel JV. Carbon-dioxide-guided vascular interventions: technique. Cardiovasc Intervent Radiol 2002;25:476–83.

14. Chao A, Major K, Kumar SR. Carbon dioxide digital subtraction angiography-assisted endovascular aortic aneurysm repair in the azotemic patient. J Vasc Surg 2007;45:451–8.

15. Criado E, Kabbani L, Cho K. Catheter-less angiography for endovascular aortic aneurysm repair: a new application of carbon dioxide as a contrast agent. J Vasc Surg 2008;48:527–34.

16. Shifrin EG, Plich WB, Verstandig A, et al. Cerebral angiography with gaseous carbon dioxide CO_2. J Cardiovasc Surg 1990;31:603–6.

17. Dimakakos PB, Stefanopoulos T, Doufas AG, et al. The cerebral effects of carbon dioxide during digital subtraction angiography in the aortic arch and its branches in rabbits. AJNR Am J Neuroradiol 1998; 19:261–6.

18. Lambert CR, deMarchena EJ, Bikkina M, et al. Effects of intracoronary carbon dioxide on left ventricular function in swine. Clin Cardiol 1996;19:461–5.

Nephrogenic Systemic Fibrosis: History and Epidemiology

Henrik S. Thomsen, MD[a,b],*

KEYWORDS

- Gadolinium based contrast media
- Nephrogenic systemic fibrosis • Epidemiology
- Prevalence • Adverse reactions

In the late 1970s and early 1980s, it was believed that the excellent soft-tissue contrast obtained using MRI technology would obviate the need for the use of contrast agents, making the procedure completely noninvasive. However, things turned out differently, and currently up to 50% of all MRI examinations worldwide are performed using contrast agents, either an extracellular agent or an organ-specific agent.

The extracellular MRI contrast agents are chelates that contain the paramagnetic ion gadolinium, which strongly affects the relaxation properties of water protons, leading to changes in tissue contrast.[1-6] Gadolinium diethylene triamine pentacetic acid salt (Gd-DTPA) was the first extracellular MRI contrast agent to be introduced in clinical practice.[1] Since the introduction of Gd-DTPA in early 1988, various gadolinium chelates with different physico-chemical properties became available for clinical use.[7-9]

SAFETY OF GADOLINIUM-BASED CONTRAST AGENTS

For many years, it was believed that gadolinium-based contrast agents (Gd-CAs) were safe. This led to a liberal use of these agents. Caravan and colleagues[10] described the situation in the late 1990s:

In the rushed world of modern medicine, radiologists, technicians, and nurses often

refrain from calling the agents by their brand names, preferring instead the affectionate "gado." They trust this clear, odorless "magnetic light," one of the safest classes of drugs ever developed. Aside from the cost ($50–80/bottle) asking the nurse to "Give him some gado" is as easy as starting a saline drip or obtaining a blood sample.

In addition, Gd-CAs were used in large doses in preference to iodine-based contrast agents for contrast-enhanced radiographic examinations in patients who had reduced renal function.[11-13] However, time has shown that Gd-CAs are not without important adverse effects.[14] Currently, radiologists are aware that intravascular administration of Gd-CAs is associated with the following safety risks: (1) nephrotoxicity that may require dialysis, (2) nephrogenic systemic fibrosis (NSF), (3) anaphylactoid and anaphylactic reactions requiring immediate intervention, and (4) reactions at the injection site.[4] With the exception of NSF, comparative studies have not shown any significant difference between the six extracellular Gd-CAs regarding diagnostic efficacy[15] and occurrence of adverse reactions.[16]

NEPHROGENIC SYSTEMIC FIBROSIS

NSF was first identified in San Diego, California, in 1997, but it took another 3 years before it was reported in the peer-reviewed literature.[17] In the

[a] Department of Diagnostic Sciences, Faculty of Health Sciences, University of Copenhagen, Blegdamsvej 3B, DK-2200 Copenhagen N, Denmark
[b] Department of Diagnostic Radiology 54E2, Copenhagen University Hospital Herlev, Herlev Ringvej 75, DK-2370 Herlev, Denmark
* Corresponding author. Department of Diagnostic Radiology 54E2, Copenhagen University Hospital Herlev, Herlev Ringvej 75, DK-2370 Herlev, Denmark.
E-mail address: hentho01@heh.regionh.dk

Radiol Clin N Am 47 (2009) 827–831
doi:10.1016/j.rcl.2009.05.003

first case series of NSF, the disease was termed scleromyxedema-like cutaneous disease in renal dialysis patients. In that series of 14 patients, 12 were receiving hemodialysis, one was on peritoneal dialysis, and 1 had acute kidney injury.[17,18] Between 2000 and 2003, reports described numerous individual cases of this disease, highlighting dermatologic and pathologic findings. Between 2003 and 2006, case reports described the clinical settings of this condition, which included chronic kidney disease, hepato-renal syndrome with renal insufficiency, and acute kidney injury. Initially, this new disease was thought to affect only the skin, hence it was given the name "nephrogenic fibrosing dermopathy." After it became apparent that the disease affects multiple organs such as the liver, lungs, muscles, and heart, the term "NSF" was adopted to reflect the multisystem involvement. In up to 50% of patients, the disease is progressive and severe.[19] NSF may contribute to death by causing scarring of organs that impairs normal function, restricting effective ventilation, or restricting movement, leading to falls that may cause fractures or hemorrhage. In one study, the 18-month mortality rate was increased significantly in patients who had NSF compared with patients who did not have NSF (40% versus 16%, respectively).[20] Swaminathan and colleagues[21] showed that of 32 patients who had NSF, 10 died at a median of 112 days after diagnosis. However, in such a high-risk group, it is difficult to differentiate deaths caused by complications of the underlying disease and its treatment from those cause by NSF.

The first publications reporting an association between Gd-CAs and NSF appeared in 2006.[22,23] Since then, numerous case series and reviews have been published. As of January 1, 2009, a total of 242 peer-reviewed papers have been registered in the National Library of Medicine (PubMed) using the keywords "nephrogenic systemic fibrosis (NSF)," with a significant increase in the number of publications in the last 3 years, from 2006 to 2008 (Fig. 1).

Cases of NSF have been reported worldwide, and the disease typically affects patients who have end-stage renal disease, including those on regular dialysis treatment. The disease has no gender, race, or age preference.[24,25] The first signs of NSF may be seen within hours of exposure to Gd-CAs, but may occur as late as 3 months after exposure.[19] It has even been claimed that NSF may occur several years after exposure to a Gd-CA.[26] During the latent period, gadolinium may accumulate in tissues other than skin, particularly in the bone.[27] There is great variability in the severity of NSF, and approximately 50% of patients who have NSF have developed a severe

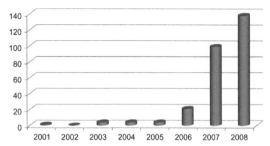

Fig. 1. Number of publications listed annually using the keywords "nephrogenic systemic fibrosis (NSF)" in the National Library of Medicine from 2000 through 2008.

form of the disease.[19] As of February 1, 2008, the peer-reviewed literature has reported that five patients had NSF in whom exposure Gd-CA could not be documented.[28] In 2009, Deng and colleagues[29] reported on seven patients who had NSF, and they were unable to identify a history of Gd-CA exposure in six of the patients, despite a thorough search of the patients' medical charts and electronic records. However, examination of specimens from three of the six patients revealed high levels of gadolinium in the affected skin of all three patients. The detected gadolinium indicates that these patients must have received a Gd-CA at some point, most likely in hospitals other than those in which the reports were conducted, because there is no other source of delivery of this metal to human tissues.

PREVALENCE

In several studies based on dermatologic, pathologic, or nephrologic registers, the prevalence of NSF after exposure to gadodiamide has been reported to be between 3% and 7% in patients who have reduced renal function.[30] The incidence of histologically proved NSF in one report of patients who had grade 5 chronic kidney disease (glomerular filtration rate <15 mL/min/1.73 m^2) who had been examined following exposure to gadodiamide was 18%.[31] The prevalence was higher after two or more injections (36%) than after a single injection (12%), indicating a cumulative effect.[31] Todd and colleagues[20] reported that 30% of patients on dialysis had developed NSF, based on a systematic examination of patients in five dialysis centers; biopsies were only taken in a few patients. In the peer-reviewed literature, the majority of cases (~85%) were associated with gadodiamide, and around 15% with gadopentetate dimeglumine. Most of the reported series of 10 patients or more were studies of patients after administration of gadodiamide, and only one report documented more than 10 patients after gadopentetate dimeglumine administration.[20] The higher prevalence of NSF in patients who had exposure to gadodiamide in comparison with patients who had exposure to gadopentetate dimeglumine is not a reflection of a higher market share; in fact, up to four to five times as many patients have received gadopentetate dimeglumine than have received gadodiamide. In a study done at four American universities, the overall incidence of NSF after exposure to gadodiamide was higher by a factor of 13 in comparison with exposure to gadopentetate dimeglumine, with incidence rates of 0.039% and 0.003% respectively.[32] The benchmark incidence of NSF was 1 in 2,913 patients who underwent gadodiamide-enhanced MRI procedures and 1 in 44,224 patients who underwent gadopentetate dimeglumine–enhanced MRI procedures ($P<.001$). The study was based on patient records from databases of dermatology, pathology, internal medicine, nephrology, transplant surgery, and radiology departments, and not on systematic examination of patients who had reduced renal function and who were exposed to a Gd-CA.

According to Medwatch, 589 people developed Gd-CA–associated NSF between 1997 and 2007; 68% of the cases were associated with gadodiamide, 26% with gadopentetate dimeglumine, and 5% with gadoversetamide. (All of these cases are associated with the administration of linear chelate Gd-CAs and, according to the European classification, the patients belonged to the high-risk group for Gd-CA inducing NSF). Three quarters of cases were from the United States, and 11% were from Denmark. The details of the Danish cases are as follows: on March 30, 2006, doctors from Copenhagen University Hospital Herlev reported 20 cases of NSF to the Danish Medicines Agency. During the following year, the number of patients increased to 30.[33] In the meantime, two hospitals (Holstebro and Hillerød) both reported that NSF had been diagnosed in one of their patients. Other hospitals denied any occurrence of NSF among their patients. Of the 32 patients, 31 had received only gadodiamide and the remaining patient received only gadopentetate dimeglumine. In January 2009, a university hospital in western Denmark announced that its staff had reviewed the records of 470 patients and found that up to 30 patients had symptoms and signs of NSF (15 patients died, 10 had biopsy-verified NSF, three are still under investigation, and in one patient NSF was considered unlikely). The prevalence of NSF in this series is similar to that reported from Herlev Hospital

(30/370). In February 2009, another university hospital in Denmark reported that it had two patients who had NSF; they were the only two patients who had end-stage renal failure who underwent magnetic resonance angiography using a nonionic linear chelate at that hospital since 2002. Thus, Denmark had, at the time this article was written, 62 patients who had NSF, of whom 43 were biopsy verified. All 62 patients received, at least once, exposure to a linear chelate Gd-CA that was one of the high-risk agents according to the European classification. There are no cases of NSF in Denmark in which the patient did not have a history of exposure to a Gd-CA. The high number of Danish cases (11% of the known NSF cases) is remarkable and not easy to explain. Denmark has only 5.5 million inhabitants and constitutes less than 1% of the population in the Western world. The medical practice does not differ from that of the other Nordic countries. The number of MRI scanners per inhabitant is less than the European average and much less than the US figure. This raises the question of whether there is a large, undiagnosed population that has NSF in other countries where gadodiamide and gadopentetate dimeglumine were the leading Gd-CAs during the first 5 years of this decade.

To date, there have been no cases of NSF after exposure to a macrocyclic agent (eg, gadoteridol, gadobutrol, or gadoterate meglumine, which are low-risk agents for NSF according to the European classification of Gd-CAs) or to the high-relaxivity agents (eg, gadobenate dimeglumine, gadofosveset trisodium, or gadotexetate sodium, which are intermediate-risk agents for NSF according to the European classification of Gd-CAs) published in the peer-reviewed literature. In all, the three macrocyclic agents have been used in nearly the same number of patients as the nonionic linear agents. A change from a nonionic linear chelate to a macrocyclic agent has eliminated occurrences of NSF from Herlev Hospital,[34] which has reported the highest number of NSF patients. (The author of this article continues to do research on this topic.)

In summary, the highest prevalence of NSF is found after exposure to gadodiamide; the incidence in patients who have end-stage renal failure, including those on dialysis, is around 10% to 15% when nonsevere cases are also included. The incidence of NSF after administration of gadopentetate dimeglumine is much lower. A few cases of NSF have been associated with gadovertisamide, but for the remaining six agents, no unconfounded cases have yet been documented in the peer-reviewed literature.

VALIDATION OF NEPHROGENIC SYSTEMIC FIBROSIS CASES

In patients who have end-stage renal failure, other skin lesions may mimic NSF. Therefore, the diagnosis of NSF should be confirmed using histologic evaluation performed by an experienced dermatopathologist in conjunction with full assessment of the clinical picture of the patient, including careful inspection of the skin lesions by an experienced clinician.[35] It is recognized that the diagnosis of NSF was excluded for some of the cases that were reported in sources outside the peer-reviewed literature, for example, in reports from the health authorities, when the cases were carefully reevaluated.

Correlation of NSF with exposure to drugs or Gd-CAs requires adequate documentation in the patient's medical records. To date, not all radiology departments have adequate registration systems for the dose and name of the contrast medium used. Sometimes, nicknames are used independent of the product administered, or a brand name continues to be used, even though a new product has been introduced. The lack of complete records has caused problems in retrospective studies performed to detect unsuspected NSF cases. It is crucially important that a record is kept of the type and dose each time an injection of a Gd-CA is given to a patient. In addition, all new cases of NSF should be reported to the appropriate national regulatory authority.[36]

Validation of NSF cases becomes even more difficult when several gadolinium products have been used. Thus, if two different Gd-CAs have been injected within one year or longer of each other, it may be impossible to determine with certainty which agent triggered the development of NSF, and the situation is described as being confounded.

SUMMARY

NSF is a severe, disabling disease. It seems to be introduced by man and seems likely to be erased by man. The first cases were diagnosed in 1997, but a correlation with exposure to Gd-CAs was not reported until 2006. Since then, the number of publications on this topic has nearly exploded. The association of NSF with an extracellular Gd-CA seems to vary according to the stability of the chelate, and the highest association was observed with gadodiamide, but no association has yet been reported in the literature with unconfounded use of macrocyclic agents.

REFERENCES

1. Nelson KL, Runge VM. Basic principles of MR contrast. Top Magn Reson Imaging 1995;7:124–36.
2. De Haën C. Conception of the first magnetic resonance imaging contrast agents: a brief history. Top Magn Reson Imaging 2001;12:221–30.
3. Wastie ML, Latief KH. Gadolinium: named after Finland's most famous chemist. Br J Radiol 2004; 77:146–7.
4. Greenen RWF, Krestin GP. Non-tissue specific extracellular MR contrast media. In: Thomsen HS, editor. Contrast media. Safety issues and ESUR guidelines. Heidelberg: Springer; 2006. p. 107–14.
5. Dawson P. Gadolinium chelates: chemistry. In: Dawson P, Cosgrove DO, Grainger RG, editors. Textbook of contrast media. Oxford: Isis Medical Media; 1999. p. 291–6.
6. Desreux JF, Gilsoul D. Chemical synthesis of paramagnetic complexes. In: Thomsen HS, Muller RN, Mattrey, editors. Trends in contrast media. Heidelberg: Springer Verlag; 1999. p. 161–9.
7. Morcos SK. Extracellular gadolinium contrast agents (Gd-CA): differences in stability. Eur J Radiol 2008; 66:175–9.
8. Idee J-M, Port M, Raynal I, et al. Clinical and biological consequences of transmetallation induced by contrast agents for magnetic resonance imaging: a review. Fundam Clin Pharmacol 2006; 20:563–76.
9. Sherry AD, Cacheris WP, Kuan K-T. Stability constants for Gd3+ binding to model DTPA-conjugates and DTPA-proteins: implications for their use as magnetic resonance contrast agents. Magn Reson Med 1988;8:180–90.
10. Caravan P, Ellison JJ, McMurry TJ, et al. Gadolinium (III) chelates and MRI agents: structure, dynamics and applications. Chem Rev 1999;99: 2293–352.
11. Hammer FD, Gofette PP, Malaise J, et al. Gadolinium dimeglumine: an alternative contrast agent for digital subtraction angiography. Eur Radiol 1999;9:128–36.
12. Spinosa DJ, Matsumoto AH, Hagspiel KD, et al. Gadolinium-based contrast agents in angiography and interventional radiology. AJR Am J Roentgenol 1999; 173:1403–9.
13. Gemmete JJ, Fortauer AR, Kazanjian S, et al. Safety of large volume gadolinium angiography [abstract]. J Vasc Interv Radiol 2001;12(part 2):S28.
14. Marzaellla L, Blank M, Gelperin K, et al. Safety risks with gadolinium-based contrast agents [letter]. J Magn Reson Imaging 2007;26:816.
15. Van der Molen AJ. Diagnostic efficacy. In: Thomsen HS, Webb JAW, editors. Contrast media: safety issues and ESUR guidelines. Heidelberg: Springer Verlag; 2009. p. 161–9.

16. Heinz-Peer G. Acute adverse reactions. In: Thomsen HS, Webb JAW, editors. Contrast media: safety issues and ESUR guidelines. Heidelberg: Springer Verlag; 2009. p. 181–4.

17. Cowper SE, Robin HS, Steinberg SM, et al. Scleromyxoedema-like cutaneous diseases in renal-dialysis patients. Lancet 2000;356:1000–1.

18. Cowper SE, Su LD, Bhawan J, et al. Nephrogenic fibrosing dermopathy. Am J Dermatopathol 2001; 23:383–93.

19. Marckmann P, Skov L, Rossen K, et al. Clinical manifestations of gadodiamide-related nephrogenic systemic fibrosis. Clin Nephrol 2008;69:161–8.

20. Todd DJ, Kagan A, Chibnik LB, et al. Cutaneous changes of nephrogenic systemic fibrosis. Predictor of early mortality and association with gadolinium exposure. Arthritis Rheum 2007;56:3433–41.

21. Swaminathan S, High WA, Ranville, et al. Cardiac and vascular metal deposition with high mortality in nephrogenic systemic fibrosis. Kidney Int 2009;73: 1413–8.

22. Grobner T. Gadolinium—a specific trigger for the development of nephrogenic fibrosing dermopathy and nephrogenic systemic fibrosis? Nephrol Dial Transplant 2006;21:1104–8.

23. Marckmann P, Skov L, Rossen K, et al. Nephrogenic systemic fibrosis: suspected causative role of gadodiamide used for contrast-enhanced magnetic resonance imaging. J Am Soc Nephrol 2006;17:2359–62.

24. Thomsen HS, Marckmann P, Logager VB. Update on nephrogenic systemic fibrosis. Magn Reson Imaging Clin N Am 2008;16:551–60.

25. Cowper SE, Rabach M, Girardi M. Clinical and histological findings in nephrogenic systemic fibrosis. Eur J Radiol 2008;66:200–7.

26. Grebe SO, Borrman M, Altenburg A, et al. Chronic inflammation and accelerated atherosclerosis as important cofactors in nephrogenic systemic fibrosis following intravenous gadolinium exposure. Clin Exp Nephrol 2008;12:403–6.

27. Thomsen HS. Is NSF only the tip of the "gadolinium toxicity" iceberg? J Magn Reson Imaging 2008;28: 284–6.

28. Broome DR. Nephrogenic systemic fibrosis associated with gadolinium based contrast agents: a summary of the medical literature reporting. Eur J Radiol 2008;6: 230–4.

29. Deng A, Bilu Martin D, Spillane J, et al. Nephrogenic systemic fibrosis with a spectrum of clinical and histopathological presentation: a disorder of aberrant dermal remodeling. J Cutan Pathol 2009; Epub.

30. Thomsen HS, Marckmann P. Extracellular Gd-CA: differences in prevalences of NSF. Eur J Radiol 2008;66:180–3.

31. Rydahl C, Thomsen HS, Marckman P. High prevalence of nephrogenic systemic fibrosis in chronic renal failure patients exposed to gadodiamide, a gadolinium(Gd)-containing magnetic resonance contrast agent. Invest Radiol 2008;43:141–4.

32. Wertman R, Altun E, Martin DR, et al. Risk of nephrogenic systemic fibrosis: evaluation of gadolinium chelate contrast agents at four American universities. Radiology 2008;248:799–806.

33. Marckmann P. An epidemic outbreak of nephrogenic systemic fibrosis in a Danish hospital. Eur J Radiol 2008;66:187–90.

34. Thomsen HS, Marckmann P, Logager VB. Enhanced computed tomography or magnetic resonance imaging: a choice between contrast medium-induced nephropathy and nephrogenic systemic fibrosis? Acta Radiol 2007;48:593–6.

35. Cowper SE. Nephrogenic systemic fibrosis. Adv Dermatol 2007;23:131–54.

36. Stenver DI. Pharmacovigilance: what to do if you see an adverse reaction and the consequences. Eur J Radiol 2008;66:184–6.

Nephrogenic Systemic Fibrosis: Clinical Picture and Treatment

Peter Marckmann, MD, DMSc[a],*, Lone Skov, MD, DMSc[b]

KEYWORDS

- Nephrogenic systemic fibrosis • Clinical picture
- Treatment • Gadolinium • Chronic kidney disease
- Renal failure • Diagnosis

Nephrogenic systemic fibrosis (NSF) was identified well before anyone knew what the cause of this feared disease is.[1,2] Today, it is beyond doubt that gadolinium (Gd)-based contrast agents (GBCA) have caused the large majority, if not all cases of NSF. The typical NSF case is characterized by a history of exposure to GBCA before the appearance of first signs of NSF and detection of Gd deposits in affected tissues.[3–6] Supporting evidence of the causal relationship between GBCA and NSF comes from ex vivo and animal studies demonstrating that Gd-salts and some GBCAs cause histologic and clinical effects resembling what is seen in NSF.[7–9] Therefore, it may be time to consider renaming NSF to what it really seems to be, which is Gd-induced systemic fibrosis. This article outlines the clinical picture and treatment possibilities of NSF.

CLINICAL PICTURE

The clinical picture of NSF is diversified.[10,11] It varies from one patient to another and it varies over time. Although the histology of deep skin biopsies most often gives important clues to the diagnosis,[12] affected skin may show panniculitis- or vasculitis-like changes in the first few weeks and nonspecific fibrosis in late stages of the disease.[13–15] Unusual clinical presentation and nonspecific histology means that it may be very hard to come to the NSF diagnosis in some patients. In practice, the diagnosis of NSF

therefore sometimes has to be based primarily on patient history of GBCA-exposures, subsequent appearance of otherwise unexplained symptoms from the skin, the limbs, or other organs, and the exclusion of relevant differential diagnoses.

This article gives a description of the classic presentation of NSF and highlights the differences between early and late manifestations of the disease. It also provides information on atypical GBCA-associated symptoms that should lead to the suspicion of NSF.

General Characteristics of Nephrogenic Systemic Fibrosis Patients

All published GBCA-associated NSF cases had acute or chronic renal insufficiency when they were exposed to GBCA.[3,12] The large majority (more than 95%) of cases had chronic kidney disease stage 5; that is, they had estimated glomerular filtration rates (eGFR) lower than 15 mL per minute per 1.73 m^2. There have been no reports of NSF cases among patients with eGFR greater than 60 mL per minute per 1.73 m^2.

The disease may affect pediatric and adult patients, but most patients are middle-aged, probably reflecting an increased use of imaging procedures for this age group.[5,16] The two sexes and different ethnicities seem to be equally affected. The primary renal disease and the duration of renal insufficiency apparently have no impact on the risk

[a] Department of Nephrology, Odense University Hospital, Soender Boulevard 29, DK-4000 Odense, Denmark
[b] Department of Dermatology KA1502, Copenhagen University Hospital Gentofte Hospital, Niels Andersens Vej 65, DK-2900 Hellerup, Denmark
* Corresponding author.
E-mail address: peter.marckmann@dadlnet.dk (P. Marckmann).

Radiol Clin N Am 47 (2009) 833–840
doi:10.1016/j.rcl.2009.05.004

of NSF. Hemodialysis patients appear to have an increased risk of NSF in its most severe form when compared with peritoneal dialysis patients and predialytic patients, probably reflecting that hemodialysis patients more frequently have the most advanced, anuric form of renal dysfunction.[17]

On the basis of published NSF case stories and cohort studies, personal clinical experiences, and retrospective scrutiny of medical records, physical examinations, and personal interviews of NSF victims, it has become clear that the course of a typical NSF case may be divided into three phases: early inflammatory, intermediate, and a late fibrotic phase (Table 1).

Early Nephrogenic Systemic Fibrosis Symptoms (Less than 2 Months After Gadolinium-Based Contrast Agent Exposure)

In the authors' experience, virtually all patients will have their initial NSF-symptoms within 2 months after the culprit GBCA exposure. The mean delay (the latent phase) from GBCA exposure to onset of clinical symptoms was 14 days in the authors' detailed study of the clinical manifestations of NSF.[10] However, some patients (around 10%) experienced their first reaction to GBCA within minutes or hours (immediate onset), whereas others had a latent phase of 4 weeks or even more (delayed onset). Similar observations have been reported by others.[18–22] According to the authors' observations, skin changes and neuropathic symptoms predominate the early phase of NSF.[10]

Skin changes
Around 90% of the patients develop an erythematous rash with or without hemorrhagic elements. The skin turns skin reddish, bluish, or brownish in color.[10,13] Some 80% of the patients have marked, nonpitting swelling of the same areas. The swellings may be misinterpreted by the clinicians as signs of over-hydration, but respond poorly to restricted fluid intake, raised dosing of diuretics, and increased dialytic ultrafiltration. The swellings are warm, relatively firm, and frequently very painful. There is an intense itching of the affected areas in most cases (70%). The skin changes are almost always localized to the limbs, primarily lower legs, in a symmetric pattern, but may extend to involve thighs and lower trunk. An estimated 10% to 20% of the patients have early involvement of hands or forearms.

Neuropathic symptoms
Almost 80% of the patients complain of pain, dysesthesia, or hyperalgesia. A minority may present with restless legs syndrome. The anatomic predilection of the neuropathy is similar to that of the skin changes. The neuropathic symptoms may be so intense that the patient becomes physically disabled. In particular, walking may become very painful.

Other symptoms
Besides skin changes and neuropathy, it is important to recognize that other body compartments and organs may be affected as part of the early phase of NSF, which includes:

  Hair: Transient, diffuse hair loss may be seen in up to 50% of the patients.
  Intestines: One-third of the patients may develop culture-negative signs of gastroenteritis with abdominal cramps, vomiting and diarrhea within the first few days after the GBCA exposure.
  Eyes: One-fifth of the patients or more may present with red eyes as sign of noninfectious conjunctivitis.
  Lungs: In the authors' material, 15% developed serious culture-negative lung symptoms, including shortness of breath, oxygen requirement, and bilateral infiltrates on chest X-ray within a few days after their GBCA exposure.

Table 1
The clinical course of GBCA-induced NSF may be divided into a latent, an early inflammatory, an intermediate, and a late fibrotic phase

Phase of NSF	Timing Relative to GBCA (Days After Exposure)	Predominant Symptoms
Latent	0–14 (range 0–60)	None
Early	14–60 (range 0–60)	Erythema, swelling, pain, itching, neuropathy
Intermediate	60–180	Mixture of early and late symptoms
Late	+180	Skin thickening and hardening, contractures, disabilities

Kidneys: Although GBCA were previously considered to have no toxic effects on kidney function, more recent reviews have concluded that nephrotoxicity may be seen with some GBCAs at a rate similar to that seen with iodine-based contrast agents.[23]

Inflammatory system: The initial phase of NSF frequently includes signs of systemic inflammation with fever, elevated C-reactive protein, elevated ferritin, anemia, and thrombocytosis or thrombocytopenia.[24,25]

The early phase may vary tremendously from one patient to the other. A minority of patients have no or very mild symptoms, whereas others may present with very dramatic symptoms from one or more organs. In case of severe early-phase symptoms, patients may suffer from associated problems, such as sleeplessness, depression, anorexia, and weight loss that may further deteriorate their situation.

In the authors' experience, some GBCA-exposed patients may develop some of the early-phase symptoms of NSF without progressing into the late and chronic phase of NSF. The authors propose that such cases might be considered and named "abortive or subclinical" NSF.

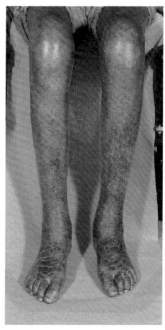

Fig. 1. Young, female hemodialysis patient with nephrogenic systemic fibrosis and classic thickening, hardening, and hyperpigmentation of the legs with flexion contractures of knees and ankles. Scaling was also prominent. The patient became dependent upon a wheelchair and died in her thirties.

Late and Chronic Nephrogenic Systemic Fibrosis Symptoms (Greater than 6 Months After Gadolinium-Based Contrast Agent Exposure)

The early-symptom complex dominates the first weeks to months, but is then gradually replaced by the late and chronic symptoms of fibrosis that are used for finally diagnosing the patient as being a NSF case. The late-symptom complex is typically stabilized 6 to 12 months after the GBCA exposure. Some case reports indicate that symptoms may appear and progress even later. In the authors' experience, late-symptom progression may indeed occur as a consequence of insufficient physiotherapy or prolonged bed rest caused by intercurrent comorbidity. The classic, hallmark signs of late stages of NSF are skin changes and contractures.[10,12]

Skin changes

The typical skin changes include islets or confluent areas of thickened and hardened dermis and subcutis, with or without sharp demarcation to the surrounding normally appearing tissues (Fig. 1). The anatomic distribution is similar to that of the early skin changes. The affected areas may have a peau d'orange appearance, and have a woody texture in the worst cases. Pinching

of the affected skin is hampered. The epidermis is typically atrophic, shiny, and hairless. However, extensive brown scaling may be seen. Hyperpigmentation (brown or dark brown) is common, but hypopigmentation is also seen. Some of the patients have discrete, superficial hemorrhages at the border of lesions on feet and toes. In the authors' cases, lower legs (from above ankles to below knees) were affected in 95%, knees and feet were affected in 50%, hands and forearms in 33%, and thighs in 25% of the NSF patients. A similar pattern of lesion distribution was reported by Cowper and colleagues.[12] The swellings that are characteristic of the early phase of NSF are virtually absent in the late phase, and the pain and itching are less prominent in most cases.

Contractures

The joint motion may be seriously reduced in anatomic regions of severe skin changes. The limited motion is primarily explained by mechanical skin forces, but it may lead to complicating joint-capsule shrinkage. Joint contractures of the ankles and knees may be seen in more than 50% of the patients, whereas wrists and elbows were affected in 33% of the authors' patients. The contractures may lead to significant disabilities, including loss of walking ability and dependence upon a wheelchair.

Although thickened, hardened skin and contractures certainly are major diagnostic criteria for NSF, it is important to acknowledge the existence of other GBCA-associated symptoms that have not received the same attention, but still may be considered part of the NSF syndrome. The other late manifestations of NSF that have marked impact on the life quality of the patient include:

Atypical skin changes: In contrast to the hardened skin of the classical NSF patient, some patients may present with sharply demarcated slack skin because of loss of dermal elastic fibers and subcutaneous atrophy. The anatomic distribution of these atypical skin changes is similar to that of classical skin changes but contractures are absent (Fig. 2).

Neuropathic symptoms: The common early neuropathic symptoms resolve to some extent in most patients. However, a considerable fraction of the patients may develop late signs of sensory and motor axonal neuropathy in the form of reduced sensibility and physical weakness of feet, legs, hands and arms. These symptoms may be disabling and limit the patients' physical performance and working ability. The early and late neurologic symptoms indicate that the fibrotic process of NSF involves the nervous tissue.[10,16]

Lungs: In parallel to the early signs of pneumonitis, respiratory insufficiency caused by lung fibrosis may occur as a late manifestation of NSF in some patients.[16]

Eyes: Yellow scleral plaques with preserved vision have been reported in various proportions of NSF patients.[12]

Muscles: Muscular atrophy of the limbs may be seen secondary to contractures, reduced mobility, axonal neuropathy, and malnutrition.

Other organs: The clinical evaluation of some NSF patients from Denmark (unpublished case reports) indicate that late NSF symptoms might also include cardiac arrhythmia and portal hypertension. However, correlating these clinical features to NSF remains speculative.

In severe cases, malnutrition is frequent and mortality is raised. Depression is also a frequent accompanying symptom of severe NSF. In spite of the multiorgan involvement, the authors have not identified any examples of reduced intellectual capacity among their NSF patients. Thus, the central nervous system seems to be spared in NSF.

The intensity and the pattern of late-NSF symptoms vary enormously among NSF cases. The authors have previously proposed a severity scoring scale of NSF that may help to distinguish mild from severe cases.[10] The scale ranges from score 0 (no symptoms) to score 4 (severely disabling symptoms causing dependence of aid or devices for common daily activities) (Table 2). In the authors' population of 22 NSF cases, 45% received a score of 4, demonstrating that a large proportion of NSF patients suffer from significant overall disability.

In general, the late-NSF symptoms can be considered stable and chronic after 12 to 24 months. Spontaneous remission of advanced chronic symptoms is unusual and cannot be expected.

RISK FACTORS

GBCA leads to NSF in only a minority of exposed patients. The reported risk of NSF after GBCA exposure ranges from 0% to 55%.[3] The large variation is partly explained by the fact that the different GBCAs are not equally risky. The nonionic linear GBCAs, in particular gadodiamide, are

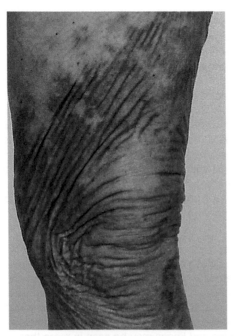

Fig. 2. Female peritoneal dialysis patient with atypical, late symptoms of nephrogenic systemic fibrosis in the form of slack skin appearance explained by elastolysis and subcutaneous atrophy.

Table 2
Severity grading (0–4) of NSF in its late phase

Grade	Clinical Presentation	Comments
0	No symptoms	NSF cases with full symptom remission
1	Mild physical, cosmetic, or neuropathic symptoms not causing any kind of disability	These cases are easily overlooked
2	Moderate physical or neuropathic symptoms limiting physical performance to some extent	May remain mis- or undiagnosed
3	Severe symptoms limiting daily physical activities (walking, bathing, shopping, and so forth)	May remain mis- or undiagnosed
4	Severely disabling symptoms causing dependence of aid or devices for common, daily activities	These cases are likely to be diagnosed and included in registry studies of NSF in contrast to patients with NSF grade 0–3

high-risk agents, whereas the cyclic agents are low-risk agents.[4,22,23,26–28] So far, there has been no scientifically verified report of NSF caused by a cyclic GBCA. Differences in study population characteristics are another reason for the large variability. Obviously, risk estimates derived from study populations with mild-to-moderate renal insufficiency will be lower than estimates derived from studies of patients with end-stage renal disease. Risk may also vary between predialytic patients, dialysis patients with residual kidney function, and anuric dialysis patients, and between patients treated with peritoneal dialysis versus hemodialysis. The risk of NSF varies even among patients with similarly poor renal function exposed to the same high-risk GBCA: some will end up as NSF victims whereas other will not. These observations illustrate that the NSF risk of an individual is modified by more factors than just type of GBCA and kidney function.

Several studies have tried to identify the risk modifiers such as acidosis[18,29] and the dose of the GBCA.[20,26,29] In the authors' case-controlled study published in 2007, it was concluded that the risk of NSF is increased with increasing cumulative GBCA exposure (ie, repeated exposures) in patients with stage 5 chronic kidney disease, and with increased serum concentration of ionized calcium and phosphate. The report also observed that high-dose erythropoietin treatment and regular hemodialysis therapy was associated with the more severe course of NSF.[17] Prince and colleagues[29] similarly found phosphate levels to modify NSF risk. Their study also suggested inflammation as a risk modifier similar to what was reported by others. Swaminathan and Shah[24] suggested a NSF promoting effect of iron

(ie, iron status and therapy). Other risk modifiers have been proposed but results have been equivocal.

In summary, GBCA exposure and advanced renal insufficiency are the two necessary causal factors in NSF pathogenesis (**Box 1**). Residual kidney function, and certain metabolic conditions, clinical states, and pharmacologic treatments seem to be risk modifiers. These risk modifiers most certainly interact mutually and with the two causal factors in a complex manner that remains to be understood. However, current best evidence suggests that states of inflammation (for example, because of malnutrition, infection, or surgery), hyperphosphatemia, and high-dose erythropoietin treatment are important promoters of NSF.

DIFFERENTIAL DIAGNOSIS

The diagnosis of NSF can be easily reached in some patients, but NSF cases with little or atypical skin manifestations might be difficult to identify. Important differential diagnoses of NSF include scleromyxoedema, morphea, systemic sclerosis, eosinophilic fasciitis, and lipodermatosclerosis. The differential diagnoses most often can be excluded from the clinical findings as described below.

Scleromyxedema

Scleromyxedema is a rare, idiopathic disease with numerous, firm and closely spaced papules of 2 mm to 3 mm in size. The skin lesions are primarily seen on hands, arms, upper trunk, neck, and face, unlike the anatomic predilection of lower legs and absent involvement of upper trunk, neck, and face in NSF. Affected areas are erythematous, with

---

Box 1
Causal factors and risk modifiers of NSF

Causal factors

Acute or chronic renal insufficiency with glomerular filtration rate below 30 mL per minute per 1.73 m² in combination with

Exposure to intravascularly administered Gd-based contrast agents

Risk modifiers associated with raised risk or increased severity of NSF

Increasingly poor renal function

High cumulated dose exposure to Gd-based contrast agents

High dose single exposure to Gd-based contrast agents

Linear nonionic > linear ionic > cyclic Gd-based contrast agents

Hyperphosphatemia

Hypercalcemia

Erythropoietin analog treatment

Inflammatory states

Risk modifiers possibly associated with raised risk of NSF

Iron status

Hypercoagulability

Surgery

Acidosis

---

scleroderma-like induration. In contrast to NSF, paraproteinemia is a frequent finding in scleromyxedema.

Morphea

Morphea is characterized by circumscribed whitish sclerotic plaques with a shiny, cicatricial center. A violaceous border may be seen in active stages. The color of the morphea elements contrasts with that of NSF elements (erythematous with or without hemorrhagic elements in the early phase, and mostly brown in late stages). In NSF, there are no specific characteristics of the center of the elements.

Systemic Sclerosis

In systemic sclerosis, the skin lesions may closely resemble those of NSF. However, systemic sclerosis typically includes marked Raynaud phenomenons, truncal and facial involvement with decreased oral aperture, significant atrophy of fingertips, and painful digital ulcerations. These findings are unusual in NSF patients. Different from NSF, systemic sclerosis is frequently characterized by marked digestive tract involvement causing dysphagia. Similar to NSF, lung fibrosis is seen. In 90% or more of systemic sclerosis patients there are antinuclear antibodies, a characteristic that is not observed with NSF.

Eosinophilic Fasciitis

Eosinophilic fasciitis initially presents as pain, erythema, warmth, swelling, and induration of the extremities. Later sclerotic changes and contractures predominate. The skin changes are typically seen over the inside of the arms and the front of the legs. The skin of the face, chest, and abdomen may also be occasionally affected. Patients with eosinophilic fasciitis have peripheral blood eosinophilia, which is not a feature of NSF.

Lipodermatosclerosis

Lipodermatosclerosis is characterized by well-circumscribed indurated, inflamed and sometimes hyperpigmented plaques and dermatitis on the lower legs in patients with longstanding venous insufficiency and stasis. The neuropathic symptoms of NSF and contractures are not seen.

In uncertain cases, information about exposure to GBCA before skin changes is important. Furthermore, skin histology would provide diagnostic clues. The histologic features of NSF are described elsewhere in this issue.

TREATMENT

The serious clinical problems of NSF patients have forced physicians dealing with these patients to institute empiric treatment. Several approaches have been tried, including systemic steroid, imatinib, chelating treatment with intravenous sodium thiosulfate, extracorporeal photopheresis, ultraviolet-A phototherapy, plasmapheresis, and more.[5,16] To the authors' knowledge, none of these treatments have been tested in controlled trials. Some of these treatments were reported to help some NSF patients in single reports, but contrasting observations were made by others. Therefore, there is still no proven curative medical treatment that can be offered to the NSF patients. However, there seems to be wide consensus that intensive physiotherapy may be of benefit in maintaining physical abilities and may even reverse lost join motion and disabilities in some cases. Symptomatic treatment with painkillers, moisturizing skin lotions, psychologic assistance, and aiding devices are important and should be considered as needed.

The only really promising solution for NSF patients is to recover their renal function. This may be obtained spontaneously in patients with acute renal failure, but requires renal transplantation in cases of chronic renal failure. Several anecdotal reports, including the authors' own experience with three transplanted NSF patients and a recent observational study indicate that significant remission of NSF symptoms may be seen after successful transplantation.[30]

SUMMARY

The objective of this article was to provide a comprehensive description of the clinical history and signs that should raise the suspicion of NSF in a patient. The NSF diagnosis may be based on history of GBCA-exposure, temporally related specific symptoms from the skin or other organs, histology of affected skin, and the exclusion of certain differential diagnoses. The present article defines early and late phases of NSF, describes early- and late-NSF symptoms, underlines the variation in NSF severity between patients, and emphasizes the existence of atypical skin changes and extra-cutaneous manifestations related to GBCA exposure in uremic patients. NSF symptoms may resolve with recovery of renal function spontaneously or as a result of transplantation.

REFERENCES

1. Cowper SE, Robin HS, Steinberg SM, et al. Scleromyxoedema-like cutaneous diseases in renal-dialysis patients. Lancet 2000;356:1000–1.
2. Daram SR, Cortese CM, Bastani B, et al. Nephrogenic fibrosing dermopathy/nephrogenic systemic fibrosis: report of a new case with literature review. Am J Kidney Dis 2005;46:754–9.
3. Marckmann P. Nephrogenic systemic fibrosis: epidemiology update. Curr Opin Nephrol Hypertens 2008;17:315–9.
4. Broome DR. Nephrogenic systemic fibrosis associated with gadolinium based contrast agents: a summary of the medical literature reporting. Eur J Radiol 2008;66:230–4.
5. Todd DJ, Kay J. Nephrogenic systemic fibrosis: an epidemic of gadolinium toxicity. Curr Rheumatol Rep 2008;10:195–204.
6. Agarwal R, Brunelli SM, Williams K, et al. Gadolinium-based contrast agents and nephrogenic systemic fibrosis: a systematic review and meta-analysis. Nephrol Dial Transplant 2009;24:856–63.
7. Varani J, DaSilva M, Warner RL, et al. Effects of gadolinium-based magnetic resonance imaging contrast agents on human skin in organ culture and human skin fibroblasts. Invest Radiol 2009;44: 74–81.
8. Grant D, Johnsen H, Juelsrud A, et al. Effects of gadolinium contrast agents in naive and nephrectomized rats: relevance to nephrogenic systemic fibrosis. Acta Radiol 2009;50:156–69.
9. Pietsch H, Lengsfeld P, Steger-Hartmann T, et al. Impact of renal impairment on long-term retention of gadolinium in the rodent skin following the administration of gadolinium-based contrast agents. Invest Radiol 2009;44:226–33.
10. Marckmann P, Skov L, Rossen K, et al. Clinical manifestation of gadodiamide-related nephrogenic systemic fibrosis. Clin Nephrol 2008;69:161–8.
11. Bangsgaard N, Marckmann P, Rossen K, et al. Nephrogenic systemic fibrosis: late skin manifestations. Arch Dermatol 2009;145:183–7.
12. Cowper SE, Rabach M, Girardi M, et al. Clinical and histological findings in nephrogenic systemic fibrosis. Eur J Radiol 2008;66:191–9.
13. Khurram M, Skov L, Rossen K, et al. Nephrogenic systemic fibrosis: a serious iatrogenic disease of renal failure patients. Scand J Urol Nephrol 2007;41:565–6.
14. Cowper SE, Su LD, Bhawan J, et al. Nephrogenic fibrosing dermopathy. Am J Dermatopathol 2001;23: 383–93.
15. Marckmann P. An epidemic outbreak of nephrogenic systemic fibrosis in a Danish hospital. Eur J Radiol 2008;66:187–90.
16. Mendoza FA, Artlett CM, Sandorfi N, et al. Description of 12 cases of nephrogenic fibrosing dermopathy and review of the literature. Semin Arthritis Rheum 2006;35:238–49.
17. Marckmann P, Skov L, Rossen K, et al. Case-control study of gadodiamide-related nephrogenic systemic fibrosis. Nephrol Dial Transplant 2007;22:3174–8.
18. Grobner T. Gadolinium—a specific trigger for the development of nephrogenic fibrosing dermopathy and nephrogenic systemic fibrosis? Nephrol Dial Transplant 2006;21:1104–8.
19. Marckmann P, Skov L, Rossen K, et al. Nephrogenic systemic fibrosis: suspected causative role of gadodiamide used for contrast-enhanced magnetic resonance imaging. J Am Soc Nephrol 2006;17:2359–62.
20. Broome DR, Girguis MS, Baron PW, et al. Gadodiamide-associated nephrogenic systemic fibrosis: why radiologists should be concerned. Am J Roentgenol 2007;188:586–92.
21. Wiginton CD, Kelly B, Oto A, et al. Gadolinium-based contrast exposure, nephrogenic systemic fibrosis, and gadolinium detection in tissue. Am J Roentgenol 2008;190:1060–8.
22. Khurana A, Runge VM, Narayanan M, et al. Nephrogenic systemic fibrosis: a review of 6 cases temporally related to gadodiamide injection (Omniscan). Invest Radiol 2007;42:139–45.

23. Penfield JG, Reilly RF Jr. What nephrologists need to know about gadolinium. Nat Clin Pract Nephrol 2007;3:654–68.
24. Swaminathan S, Shah SV. New insights into nephrogenic systemic fibrosis. J Am Soc Nephrol 2007;18:2636–43.
25. Steen H, Giannitsis E, Sommerer C, et al. Acute phase reaction to gadolinium-DTPA in dialysis patients. Nephrol Dial Transplant 2009;24:1274–7.
26. Rydahl C, Thomsen HS, Marckmann P. High prevalence of nephrogenic systemic fibrosis in chronic renal failure patients exposed to gadodiamide, a gadolinium-containing magnetic resonance contrast agent. Invest Radiol 2008;43:141–4.
27. Thomsen HS, Marckmann P. Extracellular Gd-CA: differences in prevalence of NSF. Eur J Radiol 2008;66:180–3.
28. Janus N, Launay-Vacher V, Karie S, et al. Prevalence of nephrogenic systemic fibrosis in renal insufficiency patients: results of the FINEST study. Eur J Radiol 2009. Doi:10.1016/j.ejrad.2008.11.021 [Epub ahead of print].
29. Prince MR, Zhang H, Morris M, et al. Incidence of nephrogenic systemic fibrosis at two large medical centers. Radiology 2008;248:807–16.
30. Panesar M, Banerjee S, Barone GW, et al. Clinical improvement of nephrogenic systemic fibrosis after kidney transplantation. Clin Transplant 2008;22:803–8.

Nephrogenic Systemic Fibrosis: Histology and Gadolinium Detection

Charu Thakral, MD, Jerrold L. Abraham, MD*

KEYWORDS

- Nephrogenic systemic fibrosis • Histopathology
- Gadolinium • Scanning electron microscopy
- Energy dispersive x-ray spectroscopy
- Mass spectrometry • Tissue analysis
- Secondary ion mass spectrometry

The recent and rapid emergence of nephrogenic systemic fibrosis (NSF), a systemic fibrosing disorder in patients with renal failure, has been a subject of extreme interest and debate for the past decade.[1–3] The clinical features and history are covered in another article in this issue. In 2006, Grobner[1] and Marckmann and colleagues[2] first demonstrated the association of NSF with exposure to gadolinium (Gd)-containing magnetic resonance contrast agents. The disease and its association with Gd have been identified all across the world. There have been a few reports of NSF without exposure to Gd, but any cryptic exposure to Gd cannot be definitely ruled out. A recent meta-analysis of various published case series and retrospective studies has shown a potentially causal link between the use of Gd contrast agents and the development of NSF among patients with advanced kidney disease.[3] The exact pathogenesis and mechanism of development of fibrosis still remains elusive, however. It is not yet proved if free Gd, Gd chelate complex, or the chelate itself is the cause of NSF, although the former seems most likely. The detailed pathogenesis of the tissue fibrosis is also not fully understood. It is still unclear why skin is the predominant tissue involved by this disease or if there is a specific pattern of involvement of other tissues with its progression. Specialists, including nephrologists, dermatologists, rheumatologists, pathologists, and radiologists, have been closely examining the development, with respect to the etiology, pathogenesis, and treatment of this disease.

In 2007, two laboratories (including the authors' laboratory) independently reported detection of Gd in paraffin-embedded skin biopsies of NSF tissue using scanning electron microscopy/energy dispersive x-ray spectroscopy (SEM/EDS).[4,5] To date, the authors have analyzed more than 60 paraffin-embedded skin tissues and a few autopsy cases for Gd deposition in tissues. In this article, the authors discuss in detail the histopathologic features of NSF and the methodologies of tissue Gd detection.

HISTOPATHOLOGIC FEATURES OF NEPHROGENIC SYSTEMIC FIBROSIS

Cowper and colleagues[6] first described 15 cases of a novel scleromyxedema-like fibrotic skin disease occurring in patients with renal failure who were undergoing dialysis. Since that initial report in 2000, more than 300 cases have been recognized and their histopathologic features have been characterized.

Morphologic Findings

Pathologic changes seen on routine light microscopy of biopsies of affected skin vary with disease severity, ranging from subtle changes to marked thickening of the dermis. The prominent feature of NSF is dermal fibrosis with an altered pattern of collagen bundles (Figs. 1–2). Early lesions show abundant edema fluid or mucin separating thin collagen bundles. With progression of disease, collagen bundles become thicker. The

Department of Pathology, State University of New York, Upstate Medical University, Syracuse, NY 13210, USA
* Corresponding author.
E-mail address: abrahamj@upstate.edu (J.L. Abraham).

Radiol Clin N Am 47 (2009) 841–853
doi:10.1016/j.rcl.2009.06.005

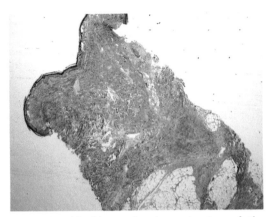

Fig. 1. NSF skin biopsy showing extension of the fibrotic process involving the subcutaneous septa between the lobules of adipose tissue.

clefts surrounding collagen bundles are present in all stages, and there is no significant inflammation. Characteristically, there are an increased number of dermal spindle cells, or fibrocytes. The fibrocytes are bland spindle cells with tapered nuclei and indistinct cell membranes. No nuclear irregularities or mitoses are noted. The fibrocytes are distributed between the collagen strands, generally parallel to their predominant direction. Mucin and refractile elastic fibers can also be identified. In advanced lesions, fibrocytes and elastic fibers are sandwiched between thick collagen bundles.[7]

In NSF, the epidermis is frequently unaffected. Some examples may show atrophy or hyperkeratosis. The entire dermis is commonly involved, with increased fibrocytes, collagen, mucin, and elastic fibers extending through the subcutaneous tissue along the septa of fatty lobules (Fig. 3). The subcutaneous septa are markedly thickened by fibrotic tissue, yielding a microlobular architecture. The fibrotic process may extend through the fascia into the underlying skeletal muscle, which becomes atrophic. Certain variations in histologic features may be noted. Some cases show abundant histiocytes or multinucleated giant cells. The authors have seen some cases with high cellularity consisting of a large number of mononuclear and multinucleated histiocytes. These rather small

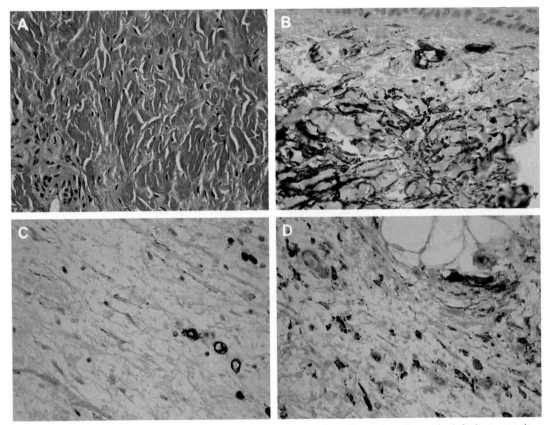

Fig. 2. (A) Dense dermal fibrosis with paler elastic fibers seen amidst collagen bundles with clefts between them (hematoxylin-eosin). Immunohistochemical stain shows (B) abundant CD34+ cells in dermis, (C) mixed CD34+ fibrocytes and (D) CD68+ macrophages in fibrotic subcutaneous septum.

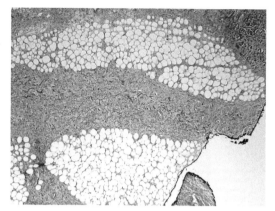

Fig. 3. Cellular fibrotic subcutaneous septum.

multinucleated cells resemble osteoclasts. It is not clear if such changes are sporadic or represent a part of the spectrum of changes seen in NSF. There is a possibility that various profibrotic cytokines, including interleukin-1 (IL-1) and transforming growth factor-β1 (TGF-β1), are released from these histiocytes, and hence promote fibrosis. Jimenez and colleagues[8] studied nine cases of severe fibrotic disease occurring in the setting of end-stage renal disease and found a marked increase in TGF-β1 mRNA levels diffusely distributed throughout the skin and fascia. All these cases also showed a marked accumulation of histiocytes or dendritic cells.

Calcification has been described in some cases as a feature of NSF.[9] It can be seen in and around thickened collagen or elastic fibers or occasionally in histiocytes. Calcification around the basement membrane of vessel walls is not uncommon. The original description by Cowper and colleagues[9] described the dermal calcification seen in older lesions as dystrophic, but another report described the concomitant presence of metastatic calcification or calciphylaxis with typical NSF histologic findings.[10] Edsall and colleagues[10] postulated that the fibrosis and calcification in NSF might be related to the activity of TGF-β1/Smad signaling cascades. TGF-β1 can have a repressive or stimulatory effect on calcification and bone growth through regulation of the production of osteopontin and profibrinogenic proteins by TGF-β1/Smad signaling cascades. A recent report described calcification within typical NSF lesions intimately associated with aggregates of fibrocytes.[11] The investigators suggested that calcification may be intrinsic to the pathophysiology of NSF and argued against nonspecific dystrophic calcification or coincidental metastatic calcification. It is difficult to separate the calcification seen in NSF from that commonly seen in patients with renal failure. Another interesting and possibly related finding is the presence of osseous metaplasia. There have been rare reports of NSF cases being dominated by foci of osteoid deposition or calcified bone spicules.[12] Osseous foci forming on refractile elastic fibers are also notable in some cases. The authors have seen a case of NSF with long-term (8 years) follow-up that showed extensive areas of osseous metaplasia in advanced lesions. There was a gradual decrease in the number of fibrocytes and development of elastocollagenous balls with foci of osteoid deposition. It is quite likely that this may represent a late stage in the evolution of NSF. Again, various theories may explain this phenomenon. Osteoblastic differentiation of some dermal cells or mesenchymal cells in an appropriate milieu may stimulate such membranous type ossification.[12,13] TGF-β1 may also be involved in this process.

There are at least six published autopsy reports of NSF in the literature. Ting and colleagues[14] first reported a case of NSF with extensive fibrosis and calcification in the diaphragm, psoas muscle, myocardial vasculature, kidneys, and testis. Other reported findings include diffuse dural osseous metaplasia; transmural bronchiolar fibrosis; fibrous plaques of the mitral valve and sclera; and fibrosis in the pleura, pericardium, and tunica albuginea.[15] The myocardium and skeletal muscles showed infiltration of the perimysium and endomysium with fibrotic tissue and muscle fiber atrophy. Fig. 4 illustrates some of the involved tissues seen at autopsy in NSF.

Histochemical and Immunohistochemical Studies

The fibrocytes have a characteristic immunoprofile, being dually positive for CD34 and procollagen 1. The staining pattern of CD34 is membranous and often reveals a much more complex dendritic network than noted in routine histologic stains. Procollagen 1 demonstrates a perinuclear cytoplasmic staining pattern of fibrocytes that becomes more intense with progression of the disease. These cells are identified as "circulating fibrocytes" and represent bone marrow–derived mesenchymal cells.[16] Mucin stains (Alcian blue and colloidal iron) and elastic stains (Verhoeff-van Gieson) may be used to highlight interstitial mucin collections and elastic fibers, respectively. Factor XIIIa+ dendritic cells and CD68+ histiocytes (mononuclear and multinucleated) are frequently found in affected tissues (Fig. 4). The factor XIIIa–expressing dermal dendritic cells are derived from the monocyte or macrophage lineage

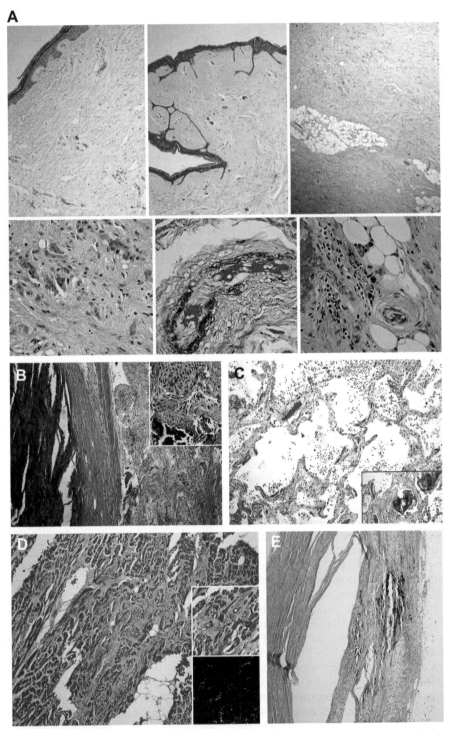

Fig. 4. (*A*) Autopsy skin, showing the variety of severity from different sites, (*top, left to right*) from minimal fibrosis and dermal edema, dense paucicellular dermal fibrosis, subcutaneous more cellular septal fibrosis. Bottom (*left to right*) showing areas of osteoclast-like multinucleated histiocytes, vascular calcification, and hemosiderin deposition. (*B*) Autopsy: fibrosis and extensive calcification of dura with clusters of meningeal cells. (*C*) Autopsy: lung with alveolar septal calcification and (*inset*) focal ossification. These findings of metastatic calcification are not specific for NSF, and currently impossible to differentiate from calciphylaxis in non-NSF patients. (*D*) Autopsy: myocardium shows interstitial fibrosis. Insets show calcification of small vessels and visualization of interstitial collagen with polarized light optics. (*E*) Autopsy: scleral plaque reveals calcification. No Gd was detectable by SEM/EDS in this heavily calcified plaque.

or from a mesenchymal origin and are increased in number in various cutaneous fibrosing lesions. Mendoza and colleagues[17] have shown coexpression of CD68 and factor XIIIa in these dendritic cells. They also noted increased numbers of these cells in early lesions of NSF. Trichrome stains for collagen and the von Kossa method for calcification are useful, especially in systemic tissues. Table 1 summarizes the histologic features, with special stains that may be used to highlight them.

Ultrastructural Findings

Electron microscopic examination of cutaneous lesions in NSF reveals dermis with abundant tortuous collagen bundles and elastic fibers, numerous spindle-shaped and elongated fibrocytes, scattered histiocytic cells, and a minimal mostly perivascular inflammatory infiltrate. In their first description of NSF, Cowper and colleagues[9] noted long thin cytoplasmic processes of spindle-shaped fibrocytes adjacent to elastic fibers and collagen bundles. Another report identified more differentiated cells with myofibroblastic characteristics, including bundles of intermediate filaments and attachment plaques in the cell periphery, indicating an ability of lesional fibroblasts to differentiate into myofibroblastic cells.[18]

DIAGNOSIS OF NEPHROGENIC SYSTEMIC FIBROSIS

None of the histologic features in NSF are definitive. The dual positivity of fibrocytes with CD34 and procollagen 1 is a helpful feature but not entirely specific. Other fibrosing lesions, including scleroderma, may also show similar dual positivity. Circulating fibrocytes have been described in a variety of conditions ranging from wound repair

to pulmonary fibrosis and asthma and are probably recruited from bone marrow to systemic tissues in response to an appropriate injury, including but not limited to endothelial damage or release of cytokines like IL-1 and TGF-β1. A clinical history of impaired renal function and negative laboratory parameters to rule out other similar fibrotic diseases are essential. It is of the utmost importance for the clinician and pathologist to have a high index of suspicion. A careful inquiry regarding all past contrast agent exposure reveals past Gd exposure in nearly all cases.

The authors believe that a full-thickness biopsy (including deep dermis and subcutaneous tissue) is essential for the diagnostic workup of suspected NSF cases. Notably, it is important to assess subcutaneous tissue for septal fibrosis. There is a probability that diagnostic features may not be detected in superficial biopsies. Sometimes, especially in late-stage lesions, the superficial dermis may show only diffuse scar-like fibrosis, although deeper areas reveal characteristic CD34+ fibrocytes. Also, calciphylaxis can be present in the same lesion and is noted only in vessels of the deep dermis and subcutaneous tissue. Certain variations, such as abundant histiocytes or elastocollagenous balls and osteoid foci, may predominate in the superficial dermis, and the typical NSF histologic features may be entirely missed in superficial biopsies. Last but not least, Gd detection is relevant to complement the histologic features or in medicolegal cases and may not be detected in superficial biopsies.

DETECTION OF GADOLINIUM

Gd is a paramagnetic ion with high toxicity. Normally, it is not found in biologic tissues.

Table 1
Histological and histochemical findings in nephrogenic systemic fibrosis skin

Histological Findings in Skin		Histochemical/ Immunohistochemical Stains
Collagen bundles with surrounding clefts	Prominent, thicker in later lesions	Trichrome
Mucin	Variable, decreases with time	Alcian blue, colloidal iron
Elastic fibers	Variable, sometimes lysis	Verhoeff-van Gieson (VVG)
Fibrocytes	Increased	CD34 and procollagen 1
Histiocytes and multinucleated giant cells/ dendritic cells	Variable	CD 68/ Factor XIIIa
Calcification	Dermal and vascular	Von kossa
Osseous metaplasia	Rare, in late stages	

Gd-containing contrast agents are discussed elsewhere in this issue.

The past few years have shown strong epidemiologic evidence of the association of Gd-containing contrast agents with the development of NSF. Furthermore, detection of Gd in tissue involved with NSF has strengthened this link.

Methods of Gadolinium Detection

Routine histology stains do not detect deposits of Gd in tissue. In general, there are two main methods for inorganic elemental analysis: microanalytic methods and mass spectrometry (MS). Both methods have been well established for detection of elements in biologic tissues. Although the principles and analytic techniques for both methods are different, they complement each other in various ways.

Microanalytic methods and gadolinium detection

Microanalysis using SEM/EDS for the detection of Gd in tissues was first reported in 1989. Elster[19] studied rat tissue specimens for tracing and localizing Gd after intracardiac injection of water-soluble Gd chelates. The tissues were flash-frozen, freeze-dried, mounted on grids, and carbon-coated for SEM/EDS analysis. With this cryopreparative method, soluble and insoluble Gd-containing materials are retained in the tissue and cannot be distinguished. Noseworthy and colleagues[20] also used a cryo-technique and were able to demonstrate Gd (presumably in intact chelate) in vessels and endothelial cells shortly after intravenous injection in rabbits. Their EDS spectra demonstrated peaks for Gd but none for phosphorus (P) or calcium (Ca). The authors used SEM/EDS to examine routine histologic tissues that are fixed in 10% formalin, processed with alcohols and xylene, and embedded in paraffin wax. The analysis of such tissues most likely detects only insoluble deposits in tissue, because compounds soluble in water or organic solvents are dissolved or washed away from the specimen. This nondestructive technique allows in situ detection of elements directly in tissues contained in the paraffin block. The direct examination on paraffin block without additional preparation or sectioning also reduces any chance of contamination from the water bath, planchettes, microtome blade, and tissue stains. The tissue in the paraffin block is scanned with SEM using the variable pressure mode (which allows examination of nonconductive samples) at an accelerating voltage of 20 kV and a working distance of 15 to 20 mm. The backscattered electron images display contrast based on atomic number differences, with higher atomic number elements seen as bright features in a darker background of organic tissues and paraffin. The electrons bombarding the tissue dislodge resident electrons in inner orbitals (K, L, and M shells) of the specimen atoms and emit characteristic x-rays (referred to as electron beam–induced x-ray fluorescence). The x-ray spectrum obtained from analyzing an individual feature (as small as 0.2 μm in diameter) reveals its elemental composition. Gd yields several characteristic L and M x-ray peaks (lines) used to confirm its presence in tissues or other specimens. The SEM/EDS system not only allows identification of the characteristic spectrum of Gd but records the precise location in the specimen. It is therefore possible to map over the electron microscopic image spatially the exact locations from which spectra of Gd were emitted. Importantly, this method also demonstrates multiple elements coassociated in a particular feature, because the entire x-ray spectrum (nominally from 0–20 kV) is examined during each analysis.

In the authors' first report, they identified Gd in all four analyzed tissues from patients who had NSF.[5] Since then, their laboratory has collaborated with various investigators around the world and has analyzed more than 80 skin tissues and tissues from a few autopsies.[21] Gd was detected in tissues involved in NSF, with none detected in tissue samples from control patients (patients with normal renal function).[22] The authors found that Gd in tissue is always associated with Ca and P. Sodium (Na) is usually present and zinc or iron (Fe) has been found, less commonly, in these deposits. Examination of the EDS spectrum of chelated Gd contrast agent reveals only Gd and no P, Ca, or Na (unless the agent formulation includes added chelate combined with Ca) (Fig. 5). Location-wise, Gd deposits were identified around the basement membrane of vessels, in eccrine glands, and in fibrous tissue, in addition to being found in individual macrophages and fibrocytes.[23] There were low levels of detectable Gd in areas of elastolytic collagenous balls and none in areas of dense ossification. Interestingly, Gd was identified more in the deeper tissue and along the subcutaneous septa. This spatial distribution is the most likely explanation for lack of detection of Gd in some superficial biopsies. To quantify the amount of detectable Gd, the authors developed a novel methodology using automated feature analysis in the SEM/EDS system.[24] The operating conditions have been standardized, and this method was shown to be reproducible. This is a semiquantitative morphometric analysis of paraffin-embedded tissues with a spatial resolution of less than 1 μm. A random search of the tissue allows in situ detection of Gd

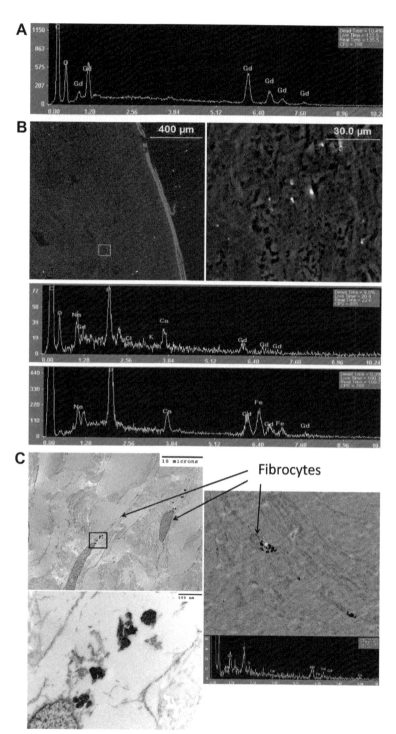

Fibrocytes

Fig. 5. (A) For comparison with the Gd deposits seen in tissues, an EDS spectrum from an Omniscan droplet is shown. Most such EDS spectra show only peaks for Gd; the one shown has a tiny peak for Ca, representing the fraction of caldiamide included as part of the Omniscan formulation. (B) (Top) SEM images of skin biopsy at ×40 magnification (left); the yellow box indicates the area shown at ×500 magnification (right), demonstrating bright features in the backscattered electron image. (Middle and Bottom) EDS spectra of individual features analyzed show Gd associated with P, Ca, and Na and also contain associated iron (bottom). (C) Transmission electron microscopy (TEM) (left: top and bottom) of skin biopsy tissue from a deparaffinized tissue block shows electron-dense deposits in the cytoplasm of fibrocytes. SEM (backscattered electron image, right) of a semithin plastic section shows the same deposits and the EDS spectrum, confirming that Gd is associated with P. In this preparation, postfixed with osmium, Ca and Na were rarely detected with the Gd-containing deposits.

and its coassociated elements; location of Gd can then be assigned to a specific site on the electron microscopic image, thus providing a distribution map (Fig. 6). The concentration of detectable Gd displayed a wide range. The authors did not find any significant correlation between the amount of detectable Gd and the amount of fibrosis. There was a definite observable difference in relative concentrations of detectable Gd and Ca with time, however. In four cases with multiple sequential biopsies over time, there was a gradual relative increase in Gd concentration and decrease in Ca concentration in Gd-containing deposits (Fig. 7).[25] The longest follow-up in one of the

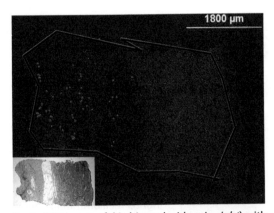

Fig. 6. SEM image of skin biopsy (epidermis, *right*) with an outline of the area analyzed and distribution of Gd-containing features (*red dots*) detected by automated analysis. (*Adapted from* Thakral C and Abraham JL. Automated scanning electron microscopy and X-ray microanalysis for in situ quantification of gadolinium deposits in skin. J Electron Microsc (Tokyo) 2007;56:181–7; with permission.)

authors' patients was 8 years. This is of concern because Gd was retained in tissue years after the last exposure. Other studies have shown similar results.[4]

Using a similar SEM/EDS system, High and colleagues[4] detected Gd in tissue of four of seven

patients who had NSF. They analyzed a single 3-μm histologic section of paraffin-embedded tissue placed on a carbon planchette. The authors have demonstrated a higher sensitivity for detection of Gd in tissues on a much thicker paraffin block compared with a thin tissue section.[24] This is a consequence of the somewhat greater volume of tissue subject to searching and EDS analysis in thicker sections or in situ in the paraffin block and may explain the relatively lesser detection ability in thinner sections. Another group studied 11 paraffin blocks from prior biopsies of seven patients diagnosed with NSF.[26] With SEM/EDS, they targeted 10 randomly selected sites (although the exact analytic protocol was not described in detail) throughout each specimen and detected Gd in six of the seven patients' skin biopsies in diseased and healthy skin.

The analytic ability of the SEM/EDS system depends on instrument and specimen factors. Instrument factors include the threshold and the time for analyzing an individual feature. In EDS spectra, the peaks of Fe can overlap somewhat with Gd. Elster[19] (using cryo-techniques) found that the upper limit of the minimum concentration of Gd was 0.005 mol/L, or approximately 0.005 mmol/g of tissue. The detection limit for the authors' automated SEM/EDS method is

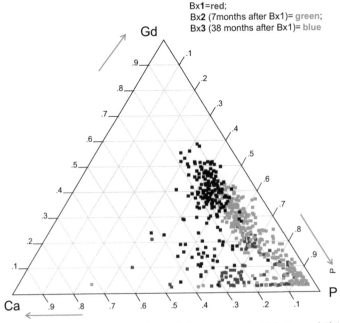

Fig. 7. Ternary plot presents the relative concentrations of three elements (Gd, Ca, and P) in individual features detected in three biopsies of a patient with NSF. This display clearly reveals the varying proportions of these elements in the different biopsies, and the increase in relative Gd concentration over 3 years, with no intervening exposure to Gd. (*From* Abraham JL, Thakral C. Tissue distribution and kinetics of gadolinium and nephrogenic systemic fibrosis. Eur J Radiol 2008;66:204; with permission.)

approximately a single feature 0.2 μm in diameter having 0.1% to 1.0% Gd by weight in a given area probed by the electron beam (the mass of Gd in such a feature would be on the order of 10^{-15} g). The smaller Gd-containing deposits or locally lower concentration Gd-containing deposits cannot be detected. The specimen factors include the concentration and distribution of Gd in the sampled tissues. The automated SEM/EDS method uses a random microanalysis of tissue. As previously noted, the authors detected Gd more in deeper tissues; thus, sampling error (eg, a superficial biopsy) may underestimate or completely miss the presence of Gd.

In most NSF cases, the microanalytic SEM/EDS system can detect Gd qualitatively and semiquantitatively. This technique does not, however, differentiate among the various chemical states of Gd; whether it is in the chelated, elemental, or ionic state cannot be definitely determined. Nevertheless, based on the known pharmacokinetics of Gd chelates, it can be presumed that detected Gd in fixed and processed tissues is in the unchelated form. Gd chelates are water soluble, and (except for special cryo-preparative techniques) the tissue examined with the SEM/EDS system has undergone processing with water, alcohols, and xylene, most likely washing out the soluble chelates and detecting only remaining insoluble unchelated Gd forms.

A more difficult microanalytic technique uses energy-filtered transmission electron microscopy (TEM) with electron energy loss spectroscopy (EELS) to detect elemental composition at the ultrastructural level. This requires ultrathin sections, as for TEM, but achieves greater spatial resolution than SEM. Schroeder and colleagues[18] demonstrated Gd-containing deposits ranging from 100 to 1000 nm in diameter in various locations in dermal tissue from an NSF case. In some of these deposits, the colocalization of Fe was also demonstrated using electron spectroscopic imaging. Colocalization of Ca or P with Gd was not reported, but detection of P and Ca is more difficult with EELS than with EDS analysis. This method searches a much smaller volume of tissue than SEM of much thicker specimens; thus, deposits of interest must be present at a high enough concentration for analysis to be successful.

Mass spectrometry and gadolinium detection
Another analytic technique that is widely popular is MS. It allows identification of the chemical composition of a specimen by sorting of gaseous ions in electric and magnetic fields according to their mass-to-charge ratios. Considered as "gold standards" for quantitative elemental analysis, these techniques are, however, tissue destructive. The tissue specimens must first be homogenized, digested, or vaporized before being analyzed by the inductively coupled plasma (ICP) or high-performance liquid chromatography (HPLC) instrument. The result is in mass of individual elements, but associations among elements that may have been combined or associated in vivo are not measurable with this method.

ICP-MS is an extremely sensitive MS method used for detection of Gd in tissues. High and colleagues[27] used this technique to quantify the amount of Gd detected in NSF tissues. Several thick sections (30 μm) of tissue cut from the paraffin block are deparaffinized, and their dry weight is measured. The ions in an acid-digested sample are extracted from plasma, passed through a quadruple, and separated on the basis of their mass-to-charge ratio. A detector receives an ion signal proportional to the concentration. Total Gd ions are monitored at the dual masses of ^{158}Gd and ^{160}Gd. Micrograms of Gd per gram of dry tissue is then calculated by dividing the mass of Gd recovered by the total mass of deparaffinized tissue analyzed. A wide range of Gd concentrations has been detected in patients who have NSF: up to 718 ppm in lesional skin, up to 5 ppm in unaffected tissue, and greater than 400 ppm in visceral organs.[28,29] Gd is not detectable in tissues from patients who have not received Gd-containing contrast agents.

In a study to assess the relations between clinical parameters and the amount of detected Gd, Khurana and colleagues[28] examined six patients who had NSF and five controls, including two with exposure to Gd. Gd levels were determined using ICP-MS. The mean Gd level detected in the affected tissue of patients who had NSF was 320.1 μg/g, and the control group demonstrated essentially no appreciable Gd in tissue. Correlation existed between higher tissue levels of Gd and younger age, lower body weight, reduced corrected serum Ca levels, and lower doses of erythropoietin. This observation may be supported by other studies that have reported an association between the development of NSF and the total dose of Gd-containing contrast agents administered.[30,31] There are discrepant results in association with serum Ca levels. Some investigators report a correlation between higher serum Ca levels and the development of NSF, but tissue Gd levels were inversely proportional to serum Ca levels in another study.[28,31]

White and colleagues[32] have used ICP-MS and detected Gd in bone a few days after intravenous Gd contrast agent administration, even in healthy volunteers without any skin lesions or renal insufficiency. There were low levels but detectable Gd (0.46–1.77 ppm) in bone after a single exposure of Gd at a dose of 0.1 mmol/kg. Other types of spectrometers using ICP, such as ICP atomic emission spectrometry, can detect Gd in concentrations as low as 1 µmol/L.[33] HPLC represents a less expensive (and less sensitive) alternative to the other analytic methods.[19] No doubt, SEM/EDS analysis is a less sensitive method for Gd detection than ICP-MS, but it has advantages in providing information about the coassociated elements and distribution of Gd-containing deposits in tissue.

A technique combining the sensitivity of MS and spatial distribution imaging is secondary ion MS. This instrumentation is used in research settings and has been used to trace Gd ions and isotopes experimentally.[34] The authors have used this method in NSF biopsy tissues and have shown much greater sensitivity for Gd detection in tissues also analyzed by SEM/EDS. The colocalization of Gd with Ca in specific cells seems to persist even in deposits not detectable with SEM/EDS analysis (Fig. 8).[35]

TISSUE GADOLINIUM AND DEVELOPMENT OF NEPHROGENIC SYSTEMIC FIBROSIS

With all the published and ongoing research in the development of NSF, two things are certain: a strong epidemiologic association with Gd contrast agents and the presence of Gd (irrespective of the method of detection) in tissues involved with NSF. The mechanism of development of fibrosis is far from clear at this point, however. The presence of free Gd ions is most favored; still, it is not proved to be strictly causative. Most patients with kidney disease who receive a Gd-containing contrast agent do not develop NSF; thus, evidently, there are other crucial factors that increase susceptibility to NSF. Current evidence favors a multifactorial model. There is almost a consensus that transmetallation that allows displacement of Gd by other elements resulting in free Gd^{3+} is a critical factor. Clinical studies showing a direct association with serum Ca levels support this. Free Gd released from its chelate likely forms insoluble precipitates with phosphate or hydroxide anions, and the authors' results of insoluble Gd deposits with phosphates clearly support that.[36,37] Gd has been reported in clinically and histologically unaffected tissues in patients who have NSF.[26] Although the authors did not detect Gd in skin biopsies from patients who did not have renal failure who had Gd-enhanced MR imaging studies,[23] they have

detected Gd in multiple organs from patients who had NSF and were examined at autopsy, some in areas with fibrosis and some in histologically normal tissues. In the authors' larger series of NSF cases from Denmark, there was only one biopsy from a clinically normal area and Gd was not detected.[22] The authors have recently reported a case with renal failure and Gd exposure but with clinical findings inconsistent with NSF; this showed histopathologic findings and Gd deposition in subcutaneous fibrotic septa indistinguishable from what has been seen in NSF.[38] Further, the relation between the amount of Gd detected and the severity of fibrosis in affected tissues is not yet clearly defined. The metabolism of Gd compounds suggests that Gd distributes and stores in different tissues, including liver and bone, for example.[36] Ongoing studies should further define the extent and distribution of Gd deposition in systemic tissues involved in NSF or show if there are alterations in the severity with location or any changes with progression of the disease. The evidence of Gd deposition in bone and the authors' results of a relative increase in Gd concentration compared with Ca raise more questions. In fact, one wonders if this long-term persistence is a reason for progression of the disease or an issue of cryptic Gd toxicity that may become better understood in the future.

There is experimental evidence that Gd can activate fibroblasts and increase collagen formation.[39] Recently, Edward (M. Edward, MD, personal communication, 2008) has extended this experimental work and demonstrated that free Gd^{3+} causes cellular injury and reaction at a much lower concentration than does gadodiamide. Several interesting theories, including recruitment of circulating fibrocytes from bone marrow or local differentiation of fibroblasts, may explain this. It is also not proved if Gd recruits fibroblasts by direct action or by means of other intermediates, such as cytokines. There is proof that histiocytes or dendritic cells release profibrotic cytokines, including TGF-β1, and may be ultimately responsible for tissue fibrosis. Because TGF-β1 is involved in the regulation of the complex process of dendritic cell maturation, it is possible that the increased expression of this growth factor is part of the response of the dendritic cells to the noxious agent, which, in this case, is Gd.

A major limitation of clinical studies of NSF is their retrospective nature and the small sample size(s). With a definite link between Gd-containing contrast agents and the development of NSF having been established, it would not be ethical to examine this association in a prospective study. The retrospective clinical data do not always allow

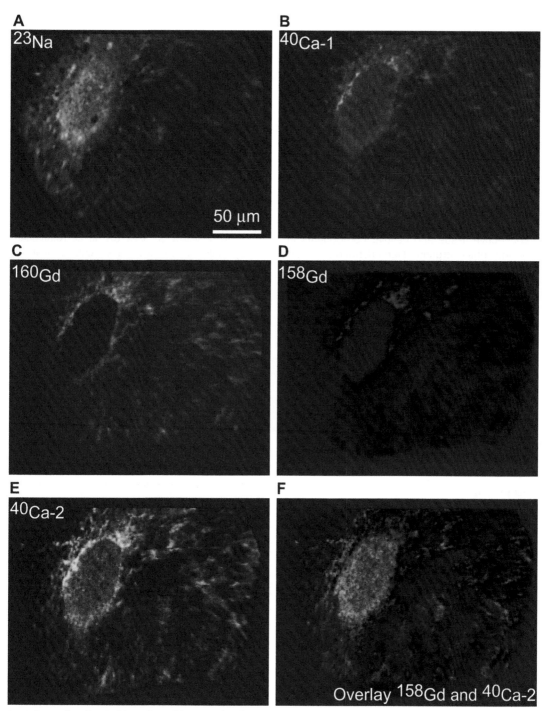

Fig. 8. Secondary ion MS imaging of human skin from a patient with NSF for Gd, Na, and Ca distributions. (A–E) Isotopic images of ^{23}Na, ^{40}Ca-1 (first Ca image), ^{160}Gd, ^{158}Gd, and ^{40}Ca-2 (second Ca image) are shown in designated panels. The ^{158}Gd and ^{40}Ca-2 images are shown in red and yellow, respectively. (F) Overlay image of Gd and Ca distributions is shown. This shows the colocalization of Gd with Ca in most of the cytoplasm but with undetectable Gd in the multinucleated giant cell. (Modified from Abraham JL, Chandra S, Thakral C, et al. SIMS imaging of gadolinium isotopes in tissue from nephrogenic systemic fibrosis patients: release of free Gd from magnetic resonance imaging contrast agents. Appl Surf Sci 2008;255:1183; with permission.)

the measurement of all the requisite clinical or laboratory parameters in a time-controlled fashion. Factors like sampling errors or biopsy depth, which are critical for accurate diagnosis and Gd determination, cannot be controlled. The development of animal models of NSF is currently an actively growing field and should yield information not available from clinical studies. This subject is beyond the scope of this review, however, and is covered elsewhere.[40,41]

SUMMARY

A review of the histopathologic findings seen in NSF cases demonstrates a variety of changes in connective tissue and cellular components in skin and other organs. Demonstration of Gd in such tissues associated with the histopathologic changes supports the causal relation of release of free Gd^{3+} from chelated Gd to the development of NSF. Analysis of Gd in tissues using nondestructive (but semiquantitative) SEM/EDS is best for demonstrating the spatial distribution of Gd-containing deposits in tissues at the histologic or cytologic scale, and the association of Gd with P and Ca in such deposits, leaving as yet unresolved the complex relation between altered Ca and P metabolism in renal failure and the development of NSF. ICP-MS (a destructive methodology) is best for determining the absolute gravimetric concentration of Gd in tissues.

REFERENCES

1. Grobner T. Gadolinium—a specific trigger for the development of nephrogenic fibrosing dermopathy and nephrogenic systemic fibrosis? Nephrol Dial Transplant 2006;21:1104–8.
2. Marckmann P, Skov L, Rossen K, et al. Nephrogenic systemic fibrosis: suspected causative role of gadodiamide used for contrast-enhanced magnetic resonance imaging. J Am Soc Nephrol 2006;17: 2359–62.
3. Agarwal R, Brunelli SM, Williams K, et al. Gadolinium-based contrast agents and nephrogenic systemic fibrosis: a systematic review and meta-analysis. Nephrol Dial Transplant 2009;24:856–63.
4. High WA, Ayers RA, Chandler J, et al. Gadolinium is detectable within the tissue of patients with nephrogenic systemic fibrosis. J Am Acad Dermatol 2007; 56:21–6.
5. Boyd AS, Zic JA, Abraham JL. Gadolinium deposition in nephrogenic fibrosing dermopathy. J Am Acad Dermatol 2007;56:27–30.
6. Cowper SE, Su LD, Bhawan J, et al. Scleromyxedema-like cutaneous diseases in renal-dialysis patients. Lancet 2000;356:1000–1.
7. Cowper SE, Rabach M, Girardi M. Clinical and histological findings in nephrogenic systemic fibrosis. Eur J Radiol 2008;66:191–9.
8. Jimenez SA, Artlett CM, Sandorfi N, et al. Dialysis-associated systemic fibrosis (nephrogenic fibrosing dermopathy): study of inflammatory cells and transforming growth factor beta1 expression in affected skin. Arthritis Rheum 2004;50:2660–6.
9. Cowper SE, Su LD, Bhawan J, et al. Nephrogenic fibrosing dermopathy. Am J Dermatopathol 2001;23: 383–93.
10. Edsall LC, English JC 3rd, Teague MW, et al. Calciphylaxis and metastatic calcification associated with nephrogenic fibrosing dermopathy. J Cutan Pathol 2004;31:247–53.
11. Song J, Volkov S, Shea CR, et al. Nephrogenic systemic fibrosis associated with stromal and vascular calcification, report of two cases. J Cutan Pathol 2008.
12. Ruiz-Genao DP, Pascual-Lopez MP, Fraga S, et al. Osseous metaplasia in the setting of nephrogenic fibrosing dermopathy. J Cutan Pathol 2005;32: 172–5.
13. Krous HF, Breisch E, Chadwick AE, et al. Nephrogenic systemic fibrosis with multiorgan involvement in a teenage male after lymphoma, Ewing's sarcoma, end-stage renal disease, and hemodialysis. Pediatr Dev Pathol 2007;10:395–402.
14. Ting WW, Stone MS, Madison KC, et al. Nephrogenic fibrosing dermopathy with systemic involvement. Arch Dermatol 2003;139:903–6.
15. Daram SR, Cortese CM, Bastani B. Nephrogenic fibrosing dermopathy/nephrogenic systemic fibrosis: report of a new case with literature review. Am J Kidney Dis 2005;46:754–9.
16. Cowper SE, Bucala R. Nephrogenic fibrosing dermopathy: suspect identified, motive unclear. Am J Dermatopathol 2003;25:358.
17. Mendoza FA, Artlett CM, Sandorfi N, et al. Description of 12 cases of nephrogenic fibrosing dermopathy and review of the literature. Semin Arthritis Rheum 2006;35:238–49.
18. Schroeder JA, Weingart C, Coras B, et al. Ultrastructural evidence of dermal gadolinium deposits in a patient with nephrogenic systemic fibrosis and end-stage renal disease. Clin J Am Soc Nephrol 2008;3:968–75
19. Elster AD. Energy-dispersive X-ray microscopy to trace gadolinium in tissues. Radiology 1989;173: 868–70.
20. Noseworthy MD, Ackerley C, Qi X, et al. Dynamic contrast enhanced magnetic resonance imaging (dMRI): verification of subcellular contrast agent location using analytical electron microscopy. Canadian Medical Physics Newsletter 2003;49:16–20.
21. Abraham JL, Thakral C, Skov L, et al. Dermal inorganic gadolinium concentrations: evidence for in

vivo transmetallation and long-term persistence in nephrogenic systemic fibrosis. Br J Dermatol 2008; 158:273–80.

22. Boyd AS, Sanyal S, Abraham JL. Gadolinium is not deposited in the skin of patients with normal renal function after exposure to gadolinium-based contrast agents. J Am Acad Dermatol 2008;59:356–8.

23. Thakral C, Abraham JL. Gadolinium-induced nephrogenic systemic fibrosis is associated with insoluble Gd deposits in tissues: in vivo transmetallation confirmed by microanalysis. J Cutan Pathol; [Epub ahead of print].

24. Thakral C, Abraham JL. Automated scanning electron microscopy and X-ray microanalysis for in situ quantification of gadolinium deposits in skin. J Electron Microsc (Tokyo) 2007;56:181–7.

25. Thakral C, Alhariri J, Abraham JL. Long-term retention of gadolinium in tissues from nephrogenic systemic fibrosis patient after multiple gadolinium-enhanced MRI scans: case report and implications. Contrast Media Mol Imaging 2007;2:199–205.

26. Wiginton CD, Kelly B, Oto A, et al. Gadolinium-based contrast exposure, nephrogenic systemic fibrosis, and gadolinium detection in tissue. AJR Am J Roentgenol 2008;190:1060–8.

27. High WA, Ayers RA, Cowper SE. Gadolinium is quantifiable within the tissue of patients with nephrogenic systemic fibrosis. J Am Acad Dermatol 2007; 56:710–2.

28. Khurana A, Greene JF Jr, High WA. Quantification of gadolinium in nephrogenic systemic fibrosis: re-examination of a reported cohort with analysis of clinical factors. J Am Acad Dermatol 2008;59:218–24.

29. Swaminathan S, High WA, Ranville J, et al. Cardiac and vascular metal deposition with high mortality in nephrogenic systemic fibrosis. Kidney Int 2008;73: 1413–8.

30. Broome DR, Girguis MS, Baron PW, et al. Gadodiamide-associated nephrogenic systemic fibrosis: why radiologists should be concerned. AJR Am J Roentgenol 2007;188:586–92.

31. Marckmann P, Skov L, Rossen K, et al. Case-control study of gadodiamide-related nephrogenic systemic fibrosis. Nephrol Dial Transplant 2007; 22:3174–8.

32. White GW, Gibby WA, Tweedle MF. Comparison of Gd(DTPA-BMA) (Omniscan) versus Gd(HP-DO3A) (ProHance) relative to gadolinium retention in human bone tissue by inductively coupled plasma mass spectroscopy. Invest Radiol 2006;41:272–8.

33. Weinmann HJ, Laniado M, Mutzel W. Pharmacokinetics of GdDTPA/dimeglumine after intravenous injection into healthy volunteers. Physiol Chem Phys Med NMR 1984;16:167–72.

34. Smith DR, Lorey DR, Chandra S. Subcellular SIMS imaging of gadolinium isotopes in human glioblastoma cells treated with a gadolinium containing MRI agent. Appl Surf Sci 2004;231–232:457–61.

35. Abraham JL, Chandra S, Thakral C, et al. SIMS imaging of gadolinium isotopes in tissue from nephrogenic systemic fibrosis patients: release of free Gd from magnetic resonance imaging contrast agents. Appl Surf Sci 2008;255:1181–4.

36. Evans CH. In: Frieden E, editor. Biochemistry of the lanthanides. New York: Plenum Press; 1990. p. 303–15.

37. Abraham JL, Thakral C. Tissue distribution and kinetics of gadolinium and nephrogenic systemic fibrosis. Eur J Radiol 2008;66:200–7.

38. Boyd AS, Sanyal S, Abraham JL. Tissue gadolinium deposition and fibrosis mimicking nephrogenic systemic fibrosis—subclinical NSF? J Am Acad Dermatol.

39. Edward M, Quinn JA, Mukherjee S, et al. Gadodiamide contrast agent 'activates' fibroblasts: a possible cause of nephrogenic systemic fibrosis. J Pathol 2008;214:584–93.

40. Pietsch H, Lengsfeld P, Jost G, et al. Long-term retention of gadolinium in the skin of rodents following the administration of gadolinium-based contrast agents. Eur Radiol 2009;19:1417–24.

41. Sieber MA, Lengsfeld P, Walter J, et al. Gadolinium-based contrast agents and their potential role in the pathogenesis of nephrogenic systemic fibrosis: the role of excess ligand. J Magn Reson Imaging 2008;27:955–62.

Involvement of Gadolinium Chelates in the Mechanism of Nephrogenic Systemic Fibrosis: An Update

Jean-Marc Idée, PharmD, MS*, Marc Port, PhD,
Anne Dencausse, PharmD, PhD, Eric Lancelot, PharmD, PhD,
Claire Corot, PharmD, PhD

KEYWORDS

- Gadolinium chelates • Thermodynamic stability
- Kinetic stability • Transmetallation
- Nephrogenic systemic fibrosis • Fibroblasts

Gadolinium chelates (GCs) are widely used to enhance the diagnostic efficacy of MR imaging for the detection and characterization of lesions and for the evaluation of perfusion and flow-related abnormalities. Two structurally distinct categories of GCs are currently marketed: (1) "macrocyclic" chelates (gadoterate, gadoteridol, or gadobutrol), in which the Gd^{3+} ion is "caged" in the preorganized cavity of the ligand, and (2) "linear" chelates (gadopentetate, gadobenate, gadodiamide, gadoversetamide, gadofosveset/MS325, and gadoxetate) (Fig. 1). GCs can also be "nonionic" (or "neutral"), in which the number of carboxyl groups is reduced to three, neutralizing the three positive charges of the Gd^{3+}, or "ionic," in which the remaining carboxyl groups are salified with meglumine or sodium.[1–3] The physicochemical features of all currently marketed GCs are shown in Table 1.

Until recently, GCs were regarded as being among the safest drugs ever introduced.[4] Allergy-like reactions to GCs, although relatively rare, do occur.[5] There is definitely no evidence that one category of GCs (linear/macrocyclic or ionic/nonionic) is associated with more reactions than another. When used in doses recommended for MR imaging, GCs seem to be nonnephrotoxic in patients with normal renal function and in patients with preexisting renal insufficiency.[6]

Since the recognition of a link between some GCs and nephrogenic systemic fibrosis (NSF) by two independent European teams in 2006,[7,8] which was later confirmed by many other studies,[9] GCs are sometimes compared with a colloidal solution of thorium, which was used as a radiocontrast agent in the period from 1930–1960 and proved to induce malignancies many years after administration.[10]

NSF is a recently described scleroderma-like disease occurring in patients with severe or end-stage renal failure.[11] The purpose of this article is to review the physicochemical properties of GCs and discuss recent issues on the possible link between these properties and the mechanism of NSF.

GADOLINIUM

Gadolinium (atomic number Z = 64) belongs to the lanthanide series of elements. Its standard atomic weight is 157.25. Gadolinium was discovered in 1880 by the Swiss chemist Jean-Charles Galissard de Marignac, isolated by the French chemist Paul-Emile Lecoq de Boisbaudran in 1886, and named after the Finnish chemist Johann Gadolin, who, in

Guerbet, Research Division, BP 57400, 95943 Roissy Charles de Gaulle cedex, France
* Corresponding author.
E-mail address: ideej@guerbet-group.com (J-M. Idée).

Radiol Clin N Am 47 (2009) 855–869
doi:10.1016/j.rcl.2009.06.006

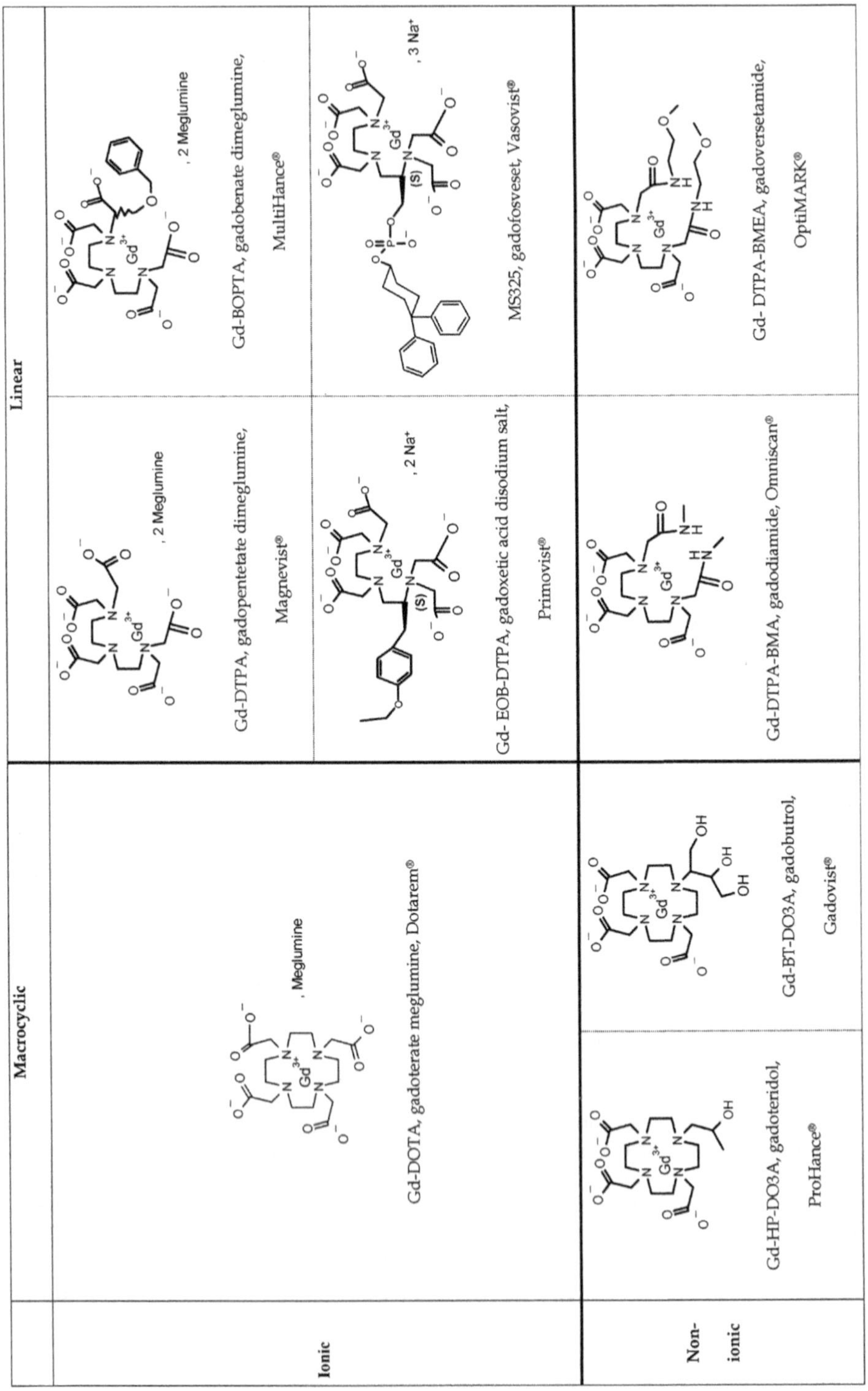

Fig. 1. Chemical structures of marketed GCs.

Table 1
General characteristics of currently marketed gadolinium chelates used for MR imaging

Name		Gd-DTPA	Gd-EOB-DTPA	Gd-BOPTA	MS325	Gd-DTPA-BMA	Gd-DTPA-BMEA	Gd-HP-DO3A	Gd-BT-DO3A	Gd-DOTA
	Acronym	Gd-DTPA	Gd-EOB-DTPA	Gd-BOPTA	MS325	Gd-DTPA-BMA	Gd-DTPA-BMEA	Gd-HP-DO3A	Gd-BT-DO3A	Gd-DOTA
	Generic Name	Gadopentetate Dimeglumine	Gadoxetic acid, Disodium Salt	Gadobenate Dimeglumine	Gadofosveset, Trisodium Salt	Gadodiamide	Gadoversetamide	Gadoteridol	Gadobutrol	Gadoterate Meglumine
	Trade Name	Magnevist	Primovist	MultiHance	Vasovist	Omniscan	OptiMARK	ProHance	Gadovist	Dotarem
Company		Bayer-Schering	Bayer-Schering	Bracco	EPIX	GE-Healthcare	Covidien	Bracco	Bayer-Schering	Guerbet
Year of first introduction		1988	2006	1997	2006	1993	2001	1992	2003	1989
Chemical structure		Open-chain	Open-chain	Open-chain	Open-chain	Open-chain	Open-chain	Macrocyclic	Macrocyclic	Macrocyclic
Charge		Di-ionic	Di-ionic	Di-ionic	Tri-ionic	Nonionic	Nonionic	Nonionic	Nonionic	Ionic
Concentration (M)		0.5	0.25	0.5	0.25	0.5	0.5	0.5	1.0	0.5
Osmolality at 37°C (mOsm/kg H_2O)		1960	688	1970	825	789	1110	630	1603	1350
Viscosity (mPa/s) at 37°C		2.9	1.19	5.3	2.06	1.4	2.0	1.3	4.96	2.0
Formulation		Free DTPA (1 mmol/L)	Ca-EOB-DTPA (trisodium salt) 1.5 mmol/L	No formulation	Fosveset (0.325 mmol/L)	Ca-DTPA-BMA (caldiamide) (Na^+ salt) (25 mmol/L)	Ca-DTPA-BMEA (Na^+ salt) (50 mmol/L)	$[Ca-HP-DO3A]_2$ (Ca^{2+} salt) 0.5 mmol/L	Ca-BT-DO3A (Na^+ salt) 1.0 mmol/L	No formulation
Hydrophilicity (log P butanol/water)		−3.16	−2.11	−2.33	−2.11	−2.13	N/A	−1.98	−2.0	−2.87
log K_{therm}		22.1	23.5	22.6	22.06	16.9	16.6	23.8	21.8	25.6
log K_{cond}		17.7	18.7	18.4	18.9	14.9	15.0	17.1	14.7	19.3
Kinetic stability[a]		Low	Medium	Medium	Medium	Low	Low	High	High	High
Approving Body		EMEA, FDA	EMEA, FDA	EMEA, FDA	EMEA, FDA	EMEA, FDA	EMEA, FDA	EMEA, FDA	EMEA	EMEA

Abbreviations: EMEA, European Agency for the Evaluation of Medicinal Products; FDA, Food and Drug Administration; N/A, not available.

[a] Low indicates long-time index (defined by Laurent and colleagues[3]) less than 0.3, medium indicates long-time index from 0.3 to 0.95, and high indicates long-time index greater than 0.95. *Data from* Idée JM, Port M, Raynal I, et al. Clinical and biological consequences of transmetallation induced by contrast agents for magnetic resonance imaging: a review. Fundam Clin Pharmacol 2006;20:563–76; and Port M, Idée JM, Medina C, et al. Efficiency, thermodynamic and kinetic stability of marketed gadolinium chelates and their possible clinical consequences: a critical review. Biometals 2008;21:469–90.

1794, analyzed the mineral gadolinite discovered at the Ytterby quarry, near Stockholm, by an amateur mineralogist.[12] In addition to its medical imaging applications related to its paramagnetic properties, gadolinium is used in electronics and optoelectronics.

To date, there is no known role of lanthanides in living systems. Free gadolinium is highly toxic.[13] The ionic radius of Gd^{3+} (107.8 pm) is close to that of Ca^{2+} (114 pm), thus making this element an inorganic blocker of voltage-gated calcium channels. Consequently, gadolinium inhibits those physiologic processes that depend on Ca^{2+} influx (eg, contraction of smooth, skeletal and cardiac muscle; transmission of nerve impulses; blood coagulation).[13] Gadolinium inhibits the activity of certain enzymes (eg, some dehydrogenases and kinases, Ca^{2+}-activated magnesium-adenosine triphosphatase, glutathione S-transferases).[14]

Gadolinium can activate the calcium-sensing receptor present on hepatocytes, kidney, thyroid and parathyroid glands, and pancreas, and, interestingly, that on fibroblasts as well.[14] Because of its biophysical similarities to calcium, gadolinium has been used to study the role of stretch-activated membrane ion channels.[14] Gadolinium is a potent and well-known inhibitor of the reticuloendothelial system.[13] Gadolinium chloride accumulates in Kupffer cells (especially in lysosomes[15]), inhibiting their phagocytic capacity and leading to their death. This effect is widely used for modeling selective depression of liver macrophages. The most pronounced toxic effects of gadolinium (and lanthanides in general) occur in the liver.[16] Gadolinium may lead to hepatocellular (and splenic) necrosis. At lower doses, it decreases cytochrome P450 activity, an effect thought to contribute to the reduction of liver injury induced by several xenobiotics, such as acetaminophen.[13] Gadolinium chloride has been found to increase activated partial thromboplastin time and prothrombin time in rats,[16] an effect probably related to its ability to inhibit Ca^{2+}-dependent reactions. Interestingly, in rats, gadolinium (at the low dose of 20 μmol/kg administered intravenously) exerts cardioprotective effects, which seem to be mediated through the JAK/STAT pathway and ATP-dependent potassium channels.[17]

After administration, lanthanides, including gadolinium, are sequestrated in the liver and skeleton. Skeletal uptake is stable, whereas hepatic uptake is labile. It remains controversial whether lanthanides associate with bone mineral or the organic matrix in bone.[18] Gadolinium has also been found to increase the expression of hepatic cytokines and several cytokine-regulated transcription factors.[13]

Free Gd^{3+} forms insoluble precipitates in the presence of hydroxide, carbonate, and phosphate anions at physiologic pH. The conditional stability constant (log K_{cond}) for gadolinium salts with phosphate is higher than with carbonate (log K_{cond}s of 22.3 and approximately 16.0, respectively[19]). It has been reported that the systemic administration of $GdCl_3$ to rats leads to mineral deposition in capillary beds and phagocytosis of minerals by macrophages.[14] Furthermore, precipitation of gadolinium may occur in physiologic salt solutions and culture media in the presence of phosphate or carbonate anions after the use of $GdCl_3$, thus leading to false-negative effects.[19] Intravenous injection of $GdCl_3$ in animals causes formation of mineral emboli in the circulation. These emboli are phagocytosed by macrophages.[14] Because of its highly acute and long-term toxicity, gadolinium must be tightly chelated by an appropriate ligand to be injected for medical imaging applications.

PHARMACOKINETICS OF GADOLINIUM CHELATES

The pharmacokinetic behavior of GCs is of paramount importance for two reasons: (1) it strongly determines their imaging profile and efficiency and (2) it depends on certain physiologic functions, notably renal function, a feature that may play a major role in the mechanism of NSF.

GCs are highly hydrophilic molecules and share pharmacokinetic characteristics similar to those of water-soluble iodinated contrast agents. They can be regarded as tracers of the extracellular water, as shown by their distribution volume, which corresponds to the human body volume of extracellular water (ie, 250–300 mL/kg). After intravenous injection, nonspecific GCs are therefore rapidly distributed in the extravascular space and excreted by glomerular filtration without any contribution from tubular secretion (elimination half-lives [$T_{1/2\beta}$s] are in the range of 1.5 hours in healthy volunteers, and almost all the injected dose is recovered in urine within 24 hours). GCs do not undergo any metabolic transformation and are eliminated unchanged.[20]

For most GCs, hepatic excretion is negligible.[20] Because of the presence of a lipophilic aromatic moiety in their structure, however, three agents (gadoxetate and gadobenate, which were developed as liver-specific compounds, and gadofosveset/MS325) bind to proteins and undergo hepatocellular uptake and partial hepatobiliary excretion (gadoxetate: 42%–51%,[21] gadobenate: 0.6–4.0%,[22] and gadofosveset: 9%[23]).

General pharmacokinetic parameters for GCs[21,23-26] are shown in **Table 2**. Classically, the pharmacokinetics of GCs are described by a two-compartment model (in which the compound is rapidly equilibrated between the plasma compartment and the extracellular compartment).[20] A three-compartment model, including the bone as a "deep" compartment (ie, a compartment associated with slow release of the compound), has been proposed for GCs.[27] In the case of compartmentalization of GCs into deep structures, such as bones, it may be speculated that pseudoequilibrium is reached locally, resulting in a gradual release of free Gd^{3+}. Consequently, more thermodynamically stable molecules should be developed to minimize the risk for free Gd^{3+} release.

The $T_{1/2\beta}$ is increased in patients with renal failure and may exceed 30 hours.[25,28] Logically, it is inversely proportional to the residual renal function.[23] No differences in terms of this phenomenon have been observed among GCs.

PHYSICOCHEMICAL PROPERTIES OF GADOLINIUM CHELATES

The effect of GCs on proton relaxation time and, consequently, their effect on the MR imaging signal depend on the large number of unpaired electrons of Gd^{3+} (n = 7). Because of its intrinsic toxicity, however, Gd^{3+} must be chelated by the administration of an appropriate ligand. Because Gd^{3+} is chelated, a thermodynamic equilibrium exists between the metal [M] (ie, Gd^{3+} in the present case), the ligand [L], and the chelate [ML]:

$$[M]+[L] \rightleftarrows [ML] \tag{1}$$

Chemists involved in the field of GCs obviously try to unbalance Equation 1 for the formation of the chelate [ML].

The stability of GCs is expressed in terms of log K_{therm}, in which K_{therm} is the thermodynamic stability constant, defined as follows:

$$K_{therm} = [ML]/[M]*[L] \tag{2}$$

In fact, a more appropriate method to compare the various agents involves the apparent thermodynamic stability constant at pH 7.4 (log K_{cond}), which considers the protonation constants of the ligand [L], and therefore describes the equilibrium at physiologic pH.[1,2]

The apparent thermodynamic stability constant is defined as follows:

$$K_{cond} = K_{therm}*[L]/L_T \tag{3}$$

in which L_T is the total concentration of the uncomplexed ligand (ie, {L + [HL] + [H_2L] +...}, in which [HL] and [H_2L] are the protonated forms of the free ligand species.

The higher the thermodynamic stability constant, the more stable is the complex and the less free toxic Gd^{3+} ion and free ligand are released.

High thermodynamic stability constants measured in water are not sufficient for in vivo stability, however.[29] Indeed, kinetic stability is another important parameter to understand the relative in vivo dissociation by describing the kinetics of dissociation of the GCs corresponding to a reaction occurring by means of spontaneous or proton-assisted dissociation of the chelate:

$$GdL \rightleftarrows Gd^{3+}+L \tag{4}$$

or the kinetics of transmetallation of the GCs by endogenous metals (particularly Ca^{2+}, Fe^{2+}, Cu^{2+}, and Zn^{2+}) according to the reaction:

$$GdL+[M]^{2+} \rightleftarrows Gd^{3+}+[ML]^- \tag{5}$$

Thermodynamic transmetallation can be defined as an exchange of metals between an

---

Table 2
Pharmacokinetic parameters of gadolinium chelates in patients with normal renal function (after intravenous administration)

Parameter	Nonspecific Chelates[a]	Gadofosveset	Gadoxetate	Gadobenate
$T_{1/2\alpha}$ (min)	3–7	N/A	N/A	28.8–36.6
$T_{1/2\beta}$ (h)	1.2–2	18.5	0.95	1.9–2.0
Vd (mL/kg)	190–280	148	210	260–280
Cl_r (mL/min/kg)	1.5–1.9	5.5	≈1.7	N/A
Cl_t (mL/min/kg)	1.6–1.9	6.6	≈3.6	1.55–1.63

Abbreviations: Cl_r, renal clearance; Cl_t, total clearance; N/A, not available; $T_{1/2\alpha}$, distribution half-life; $T_{1/2\beta}$, elimination half-life; Vd, distribution volume.
[a] Gadoterate, gadopentetate, gadoversetamide, gadodiamide, gadoteridol, gadobutrol.
Data from Refs.[21,23-26]

organometallic compound (ie, a GC in the present case) and a metal or a different organometallic compound. Transmetallation depends on the law of mass action.[1,2] The transligation phenomenon refers to the exchange of ligands.

Because the kinetics of dissociation at physiologic pH are slow, many teams have studied the rate of spontaneous or proton-assisted dissociation of GCs by measuring the half-life ($T_{1/2}$) of dissociation at pH 1.0. $T_{1/2}$ values were found to be substantially longer for macrocyclic chelates than for linear chelates.[30–32] Recently, the kinetics of dissociation of all marketed GCs at acidic pH were compared under strictly similar conditions.[2] The kinetic stability of macrocyclic chelates was classified in the following order: gadoterate > gadobutrol > gadoteridol. The $T_{1/2}$ value of all linear agents was found to be dramatically lower than that of macrocyclic GCs (Table 3).

An easy and reliable in vitro relaxometric method has been validated to evaluate the release of Gd^{3+} from GCs quantitatively in the presence of Zn^{2+} at physiologic pH.[33] As proposed by the investigators, three classes of GCs can be distinguished according to this approach: (1) macrocyclic chelates characterized by high kinetic stability; (2) ionic linear chelates for which a moderate kinetic inertia leads to significant dechelation in the presence of Zn^{2+}; and (c) nonionic linear chelates (gadodiamide and gadoversetamide), which exhibited poor kinetic stability and the highest extent of dechelation.

More recently, the stability of all GCs in human serum at 37°C was compared by high-pressure liquid chromatography coupled to a mass spectrometer. Nonionic linear complexes were shown to exhibit the lowest stability, whereas macrocyclic GCs were the most stable. Excess free ligand

in the formulation of gadodiamide and gadoversetamide delayed free Gd^{3+} release by only 2 to 3 days but did not change the dissociation rate for these molecules.[34]

Thermodynamic and kinetic stabilities must be considered together. Fig. 2 shows release of free Gd^{3+} from theoretic GCs, which differ in terms of their thermodynamic and kinetic stabilities. If sufficient time is given to the experimental system to reach equilibrium between free Gd^{3+} and its chelated form, the amount of free Gd^{3+} released depends exclusively on thermodynamic stability. If the experimental system does not allow such a thermodynamic equilibrium to be reached (eg, for pharmacokinetic reasons, such as storage in a deep compartment like bone or liver and gradual release), in other words, if earlier time points are considered, the amount of Gd3+ released depends on both the thermodynamic and kinetic stabilities of the chelate.

The higher thermodynamic and kinetic stability associated with macrocyclic agents has been confirmed by numerous in vitro and in vivo studies. The amount of Gd^{3+} internalized into tumor cells after incubation with gadodiamide was found to be approximately one order of magnitude higher than that measured with gadopentetate and the macrocyclic agents gadoterate and gadoteridol. When the experiments were performed with the commercially available formulation of gadodiamide containing the free ligand caldiamide, the amount of gadolinium detected in the cells was reduced by one half in comparison to the unformulated solution. It is worth noting that according to relaxometric and mass spectrometry measurements, the intact chelate represented only a negligible portion of total Gd species found in cells after experiments with gadodiamide.[35] It is possible that phosphate ions present in the culture medium used in these studies may have been involved in the transmetallation effect associated with gadodiamide, as suggested in human serum studies.[34] Tweedle and colleagues[36] injected radiolabeled solutions of gadopentetate, gadoterate, gadoteridol, and gadodiamide into rats and mice and measured the residual amount of ^{153}Gd at various time points up to 14 days after injection. This study clearly demonstrated that the linear chelates gadopentetate, and especially gadodiamide, led to higher amounts of residual ^{153}Gd in the whole body, liver, and femur than those of the macrocyclic chelates gadoterate and gadoteridol at late time points. These results confirmed those of a previous study[37] in which tissue distribution of radiolabeled chelates was measured after injection into mice. At 24 hours after injection, less than 0.05% of the injected dose was detected in

Table 3
Dissociation half-life ($T_{1/2}$) of all currently marketed gadolinium chelates

	$T_{1/2}$ pH = 1.0, 25°C
Gadoterate (Dotarem)	338 hours
Gadobutrol (ProHance)	3.9 hours
Gadobutrol (Gadovist)	43 hours
Linear complexes (Magnevist, Omniscan, MultiHance, Vasovist, OptiMark, Primovist)	< 5 seconds

Data from Port M, Idée JM, Medina C, et al. Efficiency, thermodynamic and kinetic stability of marketed gadolinium chelates and their possible clinical consequences: a critical review. Biometals 2008;21:469–90.

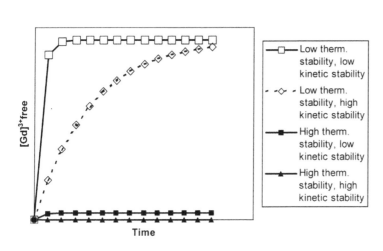

Fig. 2. Percentage of free gadolinium released by GCs of various thermodynamic (therm.) and kinetic stabilities assuming a first-order mechanism. (*Modified from* Idée JM, Port M, Medina C, et al. Possible involvement of gadolinium chelates in the pathophysiology of nephrogenic systemic fibrosis: a critical review. Toxicology 2008;248:77–88; with permission.)

the skeleton for gadoterate, whereas the amount retained in the skeleton of injected mice was higher for gadopentetate (0.30%) and gadobenate (0.22%). Gadodiamide was not tested in this study. In clinical trials in patients undergoing total hip replacement, bone tissue retention of Gd^{3+} was found to be significantly higher in patients who received gadodiamide than in those who received the macrocyclic GC gadoteridol.[38]

The difference in stability constant between Gd^{3+} and other endogenous metal ions for the same ligand is termed *selectivity*. A biospeciation model based on selectivity constants log K'_{sel} has been proposed to predict relations between thermodynamic constants and acute toxicity.[39] The aim of this model was to simulate the equilibrium that may occur after administration to rodents. Several endogenous cations (H^+, Ca^{2+}, Cu^{2+}, and Zn^{2+}) and ligands (citrate, amino acids, and serum albumin) were used in the calculations. According to this model, the selectivity constants log K'_{sel} were ordered gadodiamide > gadopentetate, which parallels the order observed for the 50% lethal dose (LD_{50}; ie, the dose that kills 50% of the test animals) for these two linear chelates. In contrast, no correlation was found between K_{therm} values and LD_{50} values. It was consequently concluded that an increase in selectivity for Gd^{3+} over endogenous body cations contributes to the high LD_{50} of gadodiamide.[39] Several important points need to be stressed, however: (1) the LD_{50} value reported with gadodiamide was obtained with divided injections, and is therefore not comparable to other published LD_{50} values for which the GC was injected as a single bolus; (2) neither iron nor phosphate was considered in the model; (3) this type of thermodynamic model does not consider the kinetic aspects related to dechelation and transmetallation; (4) as mentioned in the original article,[39] the model is not adapted to

GCs with high kinetic stability, such as gadoterate; and (5) in an in vitro transmetallation assay, the selectivity of gadodiamide for Zn^{2+} was found to be more than 10-fold lower than that calculated according to the classic model.[40]

FREE LIGAND

Because of their relatively low stability, pharmaceutic solutions of some GCs include a relatively large amount of free ligand or sodium salt of calcium complexes (see Table 1). These excipients are intended to ensure the absence of free Gd^{3+} cations in pharmaceutic solutions for the duration of their shelf lives.[1,2] According to the law of mass action (Equation 1), an excess in free ligand reduces the concentration of free Gd^{3+} and acts like a "gadolinium sponge." The least stable agents (gadodiamide and gadoversetamide) have considerably larger amounts of excess chelate (25 and 50 mmol/L; ie, 5% and 10% of the GC concentration, respectively) than the most stable agents.[1,2] There is no excess ligand in the approved formulations of gadoterate and gadobenate (see Table 1). In the case of the macrocyclic agent gadobutrol, according to its manufacturer, the calcium chelate was introduced to avoid metallic impurities that may appear during the sterilization process.[41]

HYPOTHESES FOR THE ROLE OF GADOLINIUM CHELATES IN THE MECHANISM OF NEPHROGENIC SYSTEMIC FIBROSIS

The low prevalence of the disease makes investigations on its mechanism quite difficult. Although no fully validated mechanism for NSF has been established to date, major advances have been made in the past 2 years.

In one case report,[42] the clinical condition improved after renal transplantation and subsequently relapsed after renal function was lost and dialysis was restarted. This report suggests a link between renal function and clinical signs associated with NSF. The role of renal failure might thus extend beyond delayed excretion of GCs.

Several hypotheses (which are not mutually exclusive) have been proposed to explain this disease. They are shown in **Box 1**. Although interpretation of pharmacoepidemiologic data is a complex issue,[43] it is often reported that the prevalence of NSF is higher in patients with stage 4 or 5 chronic kidney disease (CKD) who received gadodiamide than in those receiving another GC.[44–47] Because the stability of this GC is lower than that of other categories of GCs, a role has been postulated for free Gd^{3+} released associated with delayed elimination and dechelation in the body.[47–49] It is noteworthy that gadodiamide cannot be distinguished from other GCs in terms of classic physicochemical parameters, such as hydrophilicity (log P, butanol/water partition coefficient); however, being nonionic, its osmolality is lower than those of ionic GCs or agents that are nonionic and more concentrated (see **Table 1**).[2] The osmotic load with all GCs is quite low, however, because only a small volume of the contrast agent is required for most MR imaging examinations.

A threshold level of Gd^{3+} retention in tissues might be required to trigger the pathogenesis of NSF, which may explain why NSF does not affect all GC-treated patients with stage 4 or 5 CKD.[44] This level could depend on baseline renal function, the cumulative dose, and, possibly, comorbidities. It can be speculated that such a threshold level could be reached more easily in "multiple insult" animal models. The concept of threshold for NSF has also been discussed in another speculative model in which the increased burden of retained gadolinium was not regarded as playing a significant role.[65] Indeed, a quantitative serum biomarker or a validated risk stratification score would be useful to define the susceptibility of patients to NSF, and hence reduce the risk.[65] Finally, there are no published data to support a role for genetic factors.

In vivo Studies

Preclinical studies required for marketing authorization showed that the linear nonionic GCs gadodiamide[68] and gadoversetamide[69] induced skin ulceration after repeated (21 or 28 days) administration of high doses in rats. Skin lesions were observed in rats that received a maximum cumulative dose (MCD) of 18 to 19.6 mmol/kg gadodiamide administered intravenously, whereas no skin reactions were observed with an MCD of 90 mmol/kg gadoterate and gadopentetate administered intravenously.[70] These skin lesions were initially attributed to zinc deficiency.[68]

A study of repeated (20 days) injection of gadodiamide (formulated and nonformulated with excess ligand caldiamide), gadopentetate, or gadolinium-ethylenediaminetetraacetic acid (Gd-EDTA; a low-stability Gd^{3+} chelate) to rats[71] reported skin lesions, considered to be consistent with human NSF, as early as 8 days after starting nonformulated gadodiamide treatment and 20 days after starting commercial gadodiamide solution but not gadopentetate. The incidence of these macro- and microscopic lesions was also qualitatively associated with gadolinium concentrations measured in the skin. The highest gadolinium concentrations were found in the groups that received the nonformulated gadodiamide solution and the less thermodynamically stable Gd-EDTA, corresponding to the groups with the most severe skin lesions. These data support a link between released Gd^{3+} (and therefore the stability of GCs) and the development of cutaneous NSF-like lesions.

In a subsequent study, the same team reported elevation of certain cytokines (monocyte chemoattractant protein [MCP]-1 and MCP-3, macrophage inflammatory protein [MIP]-1β and MIP-2, tumor necrosis factor-α, tissue inhibitor of metalloproteinase type 1 [TIMP-1], vascular epithelial growth factor, and osteopontin) during and after repeated administrations of gadodiamide.[62] These results led the investigators to propose that in patients with severe or end-stage CKD, high serum phosphate concentrations and elevated osteopontin levels could act synergistically to trigger NSF. GCs retained in the body because of the impaired renal function would dissociate, and gadolinium may precipitate as $GdPO_4$, which is subsequently phagocytosed by macrophages. Osteopontin would play a role as a chemoattractant for immunocompetent cells, which would, in turn, activate and maintain the inflammatory pathways.[62]

Sensitized animal models with clinically relevant risk factors are obviously required. On a 5/6-nephrectomized rat model, gadodiamide and gadoversetamide administered once daily for 5 consecutive days led to higher skin gadolinium concentrations than with the ionic linear GC gadopentetate over the observation period of up to 168 days after injection.[72] After intravenous injection, the presence of gadodiamide in rat serum was dramatically prolonged in 5/6 nephrectomized rats compared with naive control animals. In the group of rats treated with the macrocyclic GC gadobutrol, the gadolinium values in the skin were even lower. This increase in the gadolinium

Box 1

Current hypotheses for the mechanism of nephrogenic systemic fibrosis (not mutually exclusive) and relevant data

- Possible involvement of an infectious agent or toxic contaminant.[50] The toxic agent seems to be gadolinium.[7,44]
- Involvement of calcineurin inhibitors (eg, cyclosporine) that are known to increase the level of transforming growth factor-β (TGFβ).[51] TGFβ may mediate the fibroblastic proliferation associated with NSF. There are no data to support this hypothesis to date; however, TGFβ was found to be associated with fibrosis in NSF skin samples.[52]
- Profibrosing effect of lanthanum, used as a phosphate binder in patients with CKD.[53] There are no data to support this hypothesis to date.
- Involvement of antiphospholipid and anticardiolipin antibodies and the human leukocyte antigen-A_2 allele.[50] There are no data to support this hypothesis to date.
- Early dermal infiltration with bone marrow-derived CD45RO+/CD34+ circulating fibrocytes in response to macrophages that have phagocytosed Gd^{3+} released from GCs.[48,49]
- Transmetallation between Gd^{3+} from less stable GCs and endogenous Fe^{3+}, with subsequent precipitation of Gd^{3+} as $GdPO_4$ associated with Fe^{3+}-induced oxidative stress (Fenton reaction).[54] Involvement of the Fenton reaction is speculative.
- Modification by Gd^{3+} of intracellular signaling through metabotropic glutamate receptors involved in skin differentiation.[55] There are no data to support this hypothesis to date.
- Immune response of the host to noxious stimuli involving dendritic cells and synthesis of TGFβ.[56]
- Erythropoietin (EPO) resistance.[57] It is unclear whether higher EPO requirements play a role in the mechanism of NSF or are the consequence of the patient's proinflammatory state.
- Metabolic acidosis as a cofactor facilitating GC dissociation.[7] This hypothesis is still being debated.[58,59]
- Activation of transglutaminases[60]
- Release of endothelin-1.[44] There are no published data to support this hypothesis to date.
- Hydrophobicity of gadodiamide facilitating entry into cells, followed by dechelation.[61] There are no data to support this hypothesis to date.
- Synergy between high phosphate levels and elevated osteopontin and chemokine levels, associated with increased microvascular permeability, leading to formation of $GdPO_4$ precipitate and uptake by macrophages.[62] This hypothesis is supported by biochemical data.[62]
- GC-induced activation of fibroblasts[63] associated with an effect of free Gd^{3+}.[64] This hypothesis is supported by data.
- Role of the timing of administration of GCs in relation to predisposing risk factors in susceptible patients.[65]
- Deleterious effect of "NSF-active" form of gadolinium (chelated form) versus "NSF-inert" form (insoluble salts, such as phosphate).[65]
- Deleterious role of angiotensin-II.[66] There are no clinical[58] or histopathologic[52] data to support this hypothesis.
- Interaction of GCs with macrophages in the extravascular space and stimulation of the expression of genes encoding profibrotic and proinflammatory cytokines in addition to the production and secretion of their corresponding products. These cytokines act on resident fibroblasts to differentiate them into myofibroblasts and stimulate their production and the release of collagens.[67] This is supported by in vitro data obtained with high concentrations of GCs.

concentration and cumulative exposure of the skin to gadolinium were inversely correlated to the stability of the GC. The skin gadolinium concentration and cumulative exposure were higher with gadodiamide than with gadoversetamide, although both compounds have the same stability and pharmacokinetics. This discrepancy may be explained by the higher free ligand concentration in the commercial solution of gadoversetamide (see Table 1). Macroscopic skin lesions were found in some of the rats treated with gadodiamide 5 days after the last administration. Interestingly, the rats with the highest skin gadolinium concentrations

also developed cutaneous NSF-like lesions.[72] Taken together, these data are consistent with facilitated dissociation of less stable GCs in renally impaired rats. In another comparative study, fibrosis of the dermis was clearly observed in gadodiamide-treated rats only.[73]

The relevance of the repeated administration model in rats was recently challenged in a study performed in naive and 5/6 nephrectomized rats receiving a high dose (5 mmol/kg intravenously for 13 doses) of formulated or nonformulated gadodiamide.[74] The researchers suggested that skin lesions found in gadodiamide-treated animals

Table 4
Histopathologic findings in patients who have nephrogenic systemic fibrosis and in rat studies

	Clinical Data[75]	Rat Data from Sieber and Colleagues[71,73] and Pietsch and Colleagues[72]	Rat Data from Grant and Colleagues[74]
Protocol	—	Euthanize 5 days after the 20th injection of 2.5 mmol/kg gadodiamide (cumulated gadodiamide dose: 50 mmol/kg)	Euthanize 1 day after the 13th dose of 5 or 10 mmol/kg gadodiamide (cumulated gadodiamide doses: 65 and 130 mmol/kg)
Histopathologic findings	Dermal fibrosis with numerous CD34+ spindle cells	Yes	No
	In early lesions, narrow collagen bundles (become thicker in more advanced disease)	Yes	No
	Procollagen-I+ fibrocytes	N/A	N/A
	Dendritic cells	Yes	N/A
	Mucin (may be virtually absent in some cases of NSF)	N/A	No
	No neutrophils and eosinophils	N/A	"Inflammation"
	Monocytes surrounding blood vessels	N/A	N/A
	Mast cells (at times)	N/A	Yes
	Epidermis not typically affected, although long-standing cases may show epidermal acanthosis	Ulceration and crust formation	Hyperkeratosis, epidermal hyperplasia, eschar, ulceration
	On occasion, loose aggregates of CD68+ histiocytes (not required to make a diagnosis of NSF)	N/A	N/A
	Calcification (within histiocytes or encrusting thickened collagen or elastic fibers)	N/A	Mineralization (nonformulated gadodiamide-treated group)

Abbreviation: N/A, not available.

were caused by pruritus and scratching and that histomorphologic changes were not consistent with those associated with human NSF.[74] As in another study,[72] gadopentetate did not induce skin lesions in this study. Table 4 compares the main histopathologic features found in patients who have NSF and in rat models with repeated administration of gadodiamide. Major discrepancies between the findings of rat studies (eg, presence or absence of CD34+ cells) and the absence of documented data on certain important markers make it difficult to draw any conclusions concerning the clinical relevance of these models. GCs and preexisting severe renal failure are necessary but not sufficient to trigger the disease. The role of cofactors, found in case-control studies, is therefore a major issue. In addition to renal insufficiency, clinical factors similar to those found in patients who have NSF may be induced in animals to increase the responsiveness to GCs, and hence the predictive value of the experimental model.

After treatment with gadopentetate, the gadolinium concentration was found to be similar to that of gadodiamide in the liver and spleen but was significantly lower in the skin, kidney, and femur of rats.[74] Several studies have shown the presence of gadolinium in skin biopsies from patients who experienced NSF after administration of a GC.[76,77] The bioanalytic techniques used in these clinical studies (and in the rat studies described previously) are unable to discriminate formally between chelated and free Gd^{3+}. Nevertheless, it seems unlikely that a water-soluble GC would persist for a long time after administration, and especially after processing of the samples in aggressive solvents and water.[76,78]

In rats, reducing the glomerular filtration rate (subtotal nephrectomy) was found to increase total skin cellularity and gadolinium retention after a single intravenous injection of gadodiamide.[79]

In Vitro Studies

By definition, in vitro studies do not allow an integrative approach of toxicity, and it is difficult to sensitize such experimental models with risk factors. These studies are essential for an in-depth understanding of the toxic effects of drugs, however. Serum from patients who have NSF has been shown to stimulate control fibroblast hyaluronan synthesis by up to 7-fold and collagen synthesis by up to 2.4-fold (comparison with control fibroblast cultures incubated with serum derived from healthy volunteers and dialysis patients not exhibiting NSF symptoms). In addition, fibroblasts exposed to gadodiamide (1.0 mM) for up to 7 days showed significant stimulation of proliferation. In this study, $GdCl_3$ (ie, "free" soluble gadolinium) had no effect on fibroblast growth, which led the investigators to propose that free Gd^{3+} may not be responsible for fibroblast growth. Gadodiamide also induced concentration-dependent stimulation of fibroblast-induced hyaluronan synthesis but did not stimulate fibroblast collagen synthesis. Finally, gadodiamide induced expression of α-smooth muscle actin staining, suggesting induction of a myofibroblast phenotype.[63] The same team subsequently reconsidered its conclusions concerning $GdCl_3$ and reported a proliferative effect for free Gd^{3+} (maximum effect at a concentration of 10 μM).[80] A proliferative effect associated with free Gd^{3+} was also found on human dermal fibroblasts in vitro at similar concentrations.[64] Interestingly, this effect was inhibited in the presence of the free ligand diethylenetriaminepentaacetic acid (10 μM), thus confirming that free Gd^{3+} actually stimulates fibroblast proliferation.[64] As expected, Gd^{3+} was found to be cytotoxic at higher concentrations. If a dose of 0.3 mmol/kg GC was administered to a patient without renal function, a maximum concentration of approximately 1.0 mM should be reached in the extracellular space. Such concentration is compatible with those of the three linear agents tested in this study. Varani and colleagues[64] found an inverse relation between GC stability and concentration required to stimulate fibroblast proliferation (active concentration gadodiamide < gadopentetate $\approx$ gadobenate < gadoteridol). GCs also increased the concentration of matrix metalloproteinase-1 (MMP-1) and TIMP-1 in the supernatant of dermal fibroblasts at the end of the 3-day culture period. With MMP-1, peak levels occurred at GC concentrations that were associated with maximal fibroblast proliferation (ie, gadodiamide [2.5–500 μM] < gadopentetate $\approx$ gadobenate [50–2500 μM] < gadoteridol [>25,000 μM]). MMP-1 (also called fibroblast collagenase-1) is a calcium-dependent zinc-containing endopeptidase involved in tissue remodeling and degradation of extracellular matrix. This multifunctional enzyme participates not only in the turnover of collagen fibrils but in the cleavage of numerous nonmatrix substrates and cell surface molecules.[81] Its substrates are collagens, proteoglycan-linked proteins, aggrecan, casein, α_1-proteinase inhibitor, and α_2-macroglobulin, for example. MMP-1 also plays a role in wound repair. Indeed, fibroblasts secrete MMP-1. This enzyme is up-regulated in fibrotic disorders.[82] From its biologic profile, it can be speculated to play a causal role in the mechanism of NSF. The increase in TIMP-1 levels may be associated with an inhibitory feedback mechanism. Finally, the GC-induced proliferative effect on fibroblasts was not associated with an increase in type I procollagen.[64]

Incubation of human monocytes with high concentrations of gadodiamide and gadopentetate (up to 50 mM over 12 or 24 hours) was recently found to be associated with marked up-regulation of numerous cytokines and growth factors. Free Gd^{3+}, tested in the form of $GdCl_3$ (up to 27 μM) had similar effects.[67] Conditioned media from these blood monocytes induced a profibrotic phenotype in normal human dermal fibroblasts.[67] In this study, no chemokines were measured and the hypothesis of the attraction of circulating fibrocytes was not addressed.

SUMMARY

There has occasionally been some confusion attributable to failure to discriminate between two complementary aspects (ie, thermodynamic and kinetic stability) to describe the stability of GCs.[1,2] **Fig. 2** illustrates release of free Gd^{3+} from theoretic GCs, which differ in terms of their thermodynamic and kinetic stabilities. The time frame of **Fig. 2** depends on pathophysiologic conditions, such as renal insufficiency, and possible storage in a deep compartment, such as bone tissue, with slow and gradual release in the body.

The mechanism of NSF remains speculative, and the exact role of GCs is still unknown. Most researchers agree that a higher prevalence of NSF is associated with the less stable linear compound gadodiamide.[43–47] This has led to speculation concerning GC dechelation in the body, associated with a subsequent proinflammatory cascade of events leading to aberrant systemic fibrosis.[47,48,62] The presence of gadolinium in skin biopsies of patients who have NSF is consistent with a role of GCs in the pathogenesis of this disease, although the currently available bioanalytic techniques are formally unable to distinguish free Gd^{3+} from its chelated form. The inverse correlation between Gd^{3+} concentrations in the skin of naive or renally impaired rats and the stability of GCs,[71,72] in addition to the occurrence of NSF-like skin lesions in rats receiving less stable GC,[71–73] suggests a causal role for free Gd^{3+}. However, gadolinium seems to be necessary but not sufficient to trigger NSF. The role of cofactors, found in case-control studies, is therefore a major issue and should be investigated, in addition to alternative hypotheses.

Because NSF is multifactorial, multiple insult models combining factors that would not, by themselves, have caused the disease seem to be more clinically relevant than studies in naive animals or "single insult" models, as pointed out in the case of iodinated contrast media–induced nephropathy models.[83]

Numerous mechanisms for NSF have been proposed to date (**Box 1**). These are not necessarily mutually exclusive. Fibrosis is a common final response to the proinflammatory effects of many drugs or substances, and future studies should focus on NSF-associated specificities. Furthermore, GCs may have proinflammatory effects, as shown with the linear agent gadopentetate, which is associated with a 10-fold increase in C-reactive protein levels in hemodialyzed patients, unlike the macrocyclic GC gadobutrol.[84] GC-induced proinflammatory effects in patients with inflammatory status may facilitate the onset of NSF.

Preclinical studies and prospective clinical trials are definitely needed to elucidate the mechanism of this major toxicologic issue and to allow better management of this devastating disease. Numerous studies are in progress.

SUMMARY

GCs are not similar in terms of stability. High kinetic stability provided by the macrocyclic structure combined with high thermodynamic stability minimizes the amount of free gadolinium released in tissue parenchymas. Although no fully validated mechanism for NSF has been established to date, major advances have been made in the past 2 years thanks to in vitro and in vivo models.

REFERENCES

1. Idée JM, Port M, Raynal I, et al. Clinical and biological consequences of transmetallation induced by contrast agents for magnetic resonance imaging: a review. Fundam Clin Pharmacol 2006;20(6): 563–76.
2. Port M, Idée JM, Medina C, et al. Efficiency, thermodynamic and kinetic stability of marketed gadolinium chelates and their possible clinical consequences: a critical review. Biometals 2008; 21(4):469–90.
3. Laurent S, Vander Elst L, Muller RN. Comparative study of the physicochemical properties of six clinical low molecular weight gadolinium contrast agents. Contrast Media Mol Imaging 2006;1(3): 128–37.

4. Caravan P, Ellison JJ, McMurry TJ, et al. Gadolinium(III) chelates as MRI contrast agents: structure, dynamics, and applications. Chem Rev 1999;99(9):2293–352.

5. Dillman JR, Ellis JH, Cohan RH, et al. Allergic-like breakthrough reactions to gadolinium contrast agents after corticosteroid and antihistamine reactions. Am J Roentgenol 2008;190(1):187–90.

6. Ledneva E, Karie S, Launay-Vacher V, et al. Renal safety of gadolinium-based contrast media in patients with chronic renal insufficiency. Radiology 2009;250(3):618–28.

7. Grobner T. Gadolinium: a specific trigger for the development of nephrogenic fibrosing dermopathy and nephrogenic systemic fibrosis? Nephrol Dial Transplant 2006;21(4):1104–8.

8. Marckmann P, Skov L, Rossen K, et al. Nephrogenic systemic fibrosis: suspected causative role of gadodiamide used for contrast-enhanced magnetic resonance imaging. J Am Soc Nephrol 2006;17(9):2359–62.

9. Agarwal R, Brunelli SM, Williams K, et al. Gadolinium-based contrast agents and nephrogenic systemic fibrosis: a systematic review and meta-analysis. Nephrol Dial Transplant 2008;24(3):856–63.

10. Wetzels JFM. Thorotrast toxicity: the safety of gadolinium compounds. Neth J Med 2007;65(8):276–8.

11. Thomsen HS, Marckmann P, Logager VB. Update on nephrogenic systemic fibrosis. Magn Reson Imaging Clin N Am 2008;16(4):551–60.

12. Wastie ML, Latief KH. Gadolinium: named after Finland's most famous chemist. Br J Radiol 2004;77(914):146–7.

13. Palasz A, Czekaj P. Toxicological and cytophysiological aspects of lanthanides action. Acta Biochim Pol 2000;47(4):1107–14.

14. Adding LC, Bannenberg GL, Gustafsson LE. Basic experimental studies and clinical aspects of gadolinium salts and chelates. Cardiovasc Drug Rev 2001;19(1):41–56.

15. Korolenko TA, Dergunova MA, Alekseenko TV, et al. Intralysosomal accumulation of gadolinium and lysosomal damage during selective depression of liver macrophages in vivo. Bull Exp Biol Med 2006;142(4):391–4.

16. Spencer AJ, Wilson SA, Batchelor J, et al. Gadolinium chloride toxicity in the rat. Toxicol Pathol 1997;25(3):245–55.

17. Nicolosi AC, Strande JL, Hsu A, et al. Gadolinium limits myocardial infarction in the rat: dose-response, temporal relations and mechanisms. J Mol Cell Cardiol 2008;44(2):345–51.

18. Evans CH. The occurrence and metabolism of lanthanides. In: Biochemistry of the lanthanides. New York: Plenum Press; 1990. p. 285–337.

19. Caldwell RA, Clemo HF, Baumgarten CM. Using gadolinium to identify stretch-activated channels. Am J Physiol 1998;275(2 Pt 1):C619–21.

20. Lorusso V, Pascolo L, Fernetti C, et al. Magnetic resonance contrast agents: from the bench to the patient. Curr Pharm Des 2005;11(31):4079–98.

21. Hamm B, Staks T, Mühler A, et al. Phase I clinical evaluation of Gd-EOB-DTPA as a hepatobiliary MR contrast agent: safety, pharmacokinetics, and MR imaging. Radiology 1995;195(3):785–92.

22. Spinazzi A, Lorusso V, Pirovano G, et-al. Safety, tolerance, biodistribution and MR imaging enhancement of the liver with gadobenate dimeglumine: results of clinical pharmacologic and pilot imaging studies in nonpatient and patient volunteers. Acad Radiol 1999;6(5):282–91.

23. Ersoy H, Rybicki FJ. Biochemical safety profiles of gadolinium-based extracellular contrast agents and nephrogenic systemic fibrosis. J Magn Reson Imaging 2007;26(5):1190–7.

24. Van Wagoner M, O'Toole M, Worah D, et al. A phase I clinical trial with gadodiamide injection, a nonionic magnetic resonance imaging enhancement agent. Invest Radiol 1991;26(11):980–6.

25. Swan SK, Lambrecht LJ, Townsend R, et al. Safety and pharmacokinetic profile of gadobenate dimeglumine in subjects with renal impairment. Invest Radiol 1999;34(7):443–8.

26. Henness S, Keating GM. Gadofosveset. Drugs 2006;66(6):851–7.

27. Hirano S, Suzuki KT. Exposure, metabolism, and toxicity of rare earths and related compounds. Environ Health Perspect 1996;104(Suppl 1):85–95.

28. Joffe P, Thomsen HS, Meusel M. Pharmacokinetics of gadodiamide injection in patients with severe renal insufficiency and patients undergoing hemodialysis or continuous ambulatory peritoneal dialysis. Acad Radiol 1998;5(7):491–502.

29. Tweedle MF, Hagan JJ, Kumar K, et al. Reaction of gadolinium chelates with endogenously available ions. Magn Reson Imaging 1991;9(3):409–15.

30. Kumar K, Chang CA, Tweedle MF. Equilibrium and kinetic studies of lanthanide complexes of macrocyclic polyamino carboxylates. Inorg Chem 1993;32(5):587–93.

31. Tweedle MF. Physicochemical properties of gadoteridol and other magnetic resonance contrast agents. Invest Radiol 1992;27(Suppl 1):S2–6.

32. Wedeking P, Kumar K, Tweedle MF. Dissociation of gadolinium chelates in mice: relationship to chemical characteristics. Magn Reson Imaging 1992;10(4):641–8.

33. Laurent S, Vander Elst L, Copoix F, et al. Stability of MRI paramagnetic contrast media. A proton relaxometric protocol for transmetallation assessment. Invest Radiol 2001;36(2):115–22.

34. Frenzel T, Lengsfeld P, Schirmer H, et al. Stability of gadolinium-based contrast agents in human serum at 37°C. Invest Radiol 2008;43(12):817–28.

35. Cabella C, Geninatti Crich S, Corpillo D, et al. Cellular labelling with Gd(III) chelates: only high

thermodynamic stabilities prevent the cells acting as "sponges" of Gd^{3+} ions. Contrast Media Mol Imaging 2006;1(1):23–9.

36. Tweedle MF, Wedeking P, Kumar K. Biodistribution of radiolabeled, formulated gadopentetate, gadoteridol, gadoterate, and gadodiamide in mice and rats. Invest Radiol 1995;30(6):372–80.

37. Harrison A, Walker CA, Pereira KA, et al. Hepatobiliary and renal excretion in mice of charged and neutral gadolinium complexes of cyclic tetra-aza-phosphinic and carboxylic acids. Magn Reson Imaging 1993;11(6):761–70.

38. White GW, Gibby WA, Tweedle MF. Comparison of Gd(DTPA-BMA) (Omniscan) versus Gd(HP-DO3A) (ProHance) relative to gadolinium retention in human bone tissue by inductively coupled mass spectroscopy. Invest Radiol 2006;41(3):272–8.

39. Cacheris WP, Quay SC, Rocklage SM. The relationship between thermodynamics and the toxicity of gadolinium complexes. Magn Reson Imaging 1990;8(4):467–81.

40. Puttagunta NR, Gibby WA, Smith GT. Human in vivo comparative study of zinc and copper transmetallation after administration of magnetic resonance imaging contrast agents. Invest Radiol 1996; 31(12):739–42.

41. Schmitt-Willich H. Stability of linear and macrocyclic gadolinium based contrast agents. Br J Radiol 2007; 80(955):581–5.

42. Goddard DS, Magee CC, Lazar AJF, et al. Nephrogenic fibrosing dermopathy with recurrence after allograft failure. J Am Acad Dermatol 2007;56(Suppl 5):S109–11.

43. Penfield JG, Reilly RF. Nephrogenic systemic fibrosis risk: is there a difference between gadolinium-based contrast agents? Semin Dial 2008; 21(2):129–34.

44. Cowper SE. Nephrogenic systemic fibrosis: a review and exploration of the role of gadolinium. Adv Dermatol 2007;23:131–54.

45. Thomsen H, Marckmann P. Extracellular Gd-CA: differences in prevalence of NSF. Eur J Radiol 2008;66(2):180–3.

46. Kanal E, Barkovich AJ, Bell C, et al. ACR guidance document for safe MR practices: 2007. Am J Roentgenol 2007;188(6):1447–74.

47. Perazella MA. Current status of gadolinium toxicity in patients with kidney disease. Clin J Am Soc Nephrol 2009;4(2):461–9.

48. Morcos SK. Nephrogenic systemic fibrosis following the administration of extracellular gadolinium-based contrast agents: is the stability of the contrast agent molecule an important factor in the pathogenesis of this condition? Br J Radiol 2007;80(950):73–6.

49. Perazella MA. Tissue deposition of gadolinium and development of NSF: a convergence of factors. Semin Dial 2008;21(2):150–4.

50. Evenepoel P, Zeegers M, Segaert S, et al. Nephrogenic fibrosing dermopathy: a novel, disabling disorder in patients with renal failure. Nephrol Dial Transplant 2004;19(2):469–73.

51. Shin GT, Khanna A, Ding R, et al. In vivo expression of transforming growth-factor-beta 1 in humans: stimulation by cyclosporine. Transplantation 1998;65(3):313–8.

52. Kelly B, Petitt M, Sanchez R. Nephrogenic systemic fibrosis is associated with transforming growth factor beta and Smad without evidence of renin-angiotensin system involvement. J Am Acad Dermatol 2008;58(6):1025–30.

53. Aime S, Canavese C, Stratta P. Advisory about gadolinium calls for caution in the treatment of uremic patients with lanthanum carbonate. Kidney Int 2007;72(9):1162–3.

54. Swaminathan S, Shah SV. New insights into nephrogenic systemic fibrosis. J Am Soc Nephrol 2007; 18(10):2636–43.

55. Othersen JB, Maize JC, Woolson RF, et al. Nephrogenic systemic fibrosis after exposure to gadolinium in patients with renal failure. Nephrol Dial Transplant 2007;22(11):3179–85.

56. Mendoza FA, Artlett CM, Sandorfi N, et al. Description of 12 cases of nephrogenic fibrosing dermopathy and review of the literature. Semin Arthritis Rheum 2006;35(4):238–49.

57. Swaminathan S, Ahmed I, McCarthy JT, et al. Nephrogenic fibrosing dermopathy and high-dose erythropoietin therapy. Ann Intern Med 2006; 145(3):234–5.

58. Marckmann P, Skov L, Rossen K. Case-control study of gadodiamide-related nephrogenic systemic fibrosis. Nephrol Dial Transplant 2007;22(11):3174–8.

59. Sadowski EA, Bennett LK, Chan MR, et al. Nephrogenic systemic fibrosis: risk factors and incidence estimation. Radiology 2007;243(1):148–57.

60. Parsons AC, Yosipovitch G, Sheehan DJ, et al. Transglutaminases: the missing link in nephrogenic systemic fibrosis. Am J Dermatopathol 2007;29(5):433–6.

61. Dawson P. Nephrogenic systemic fibrosis: possible mechanisms and imaging management strategies. J Magn Reson Imaging 2008;28(4):797–804.

62. Steger-Hartmann T, Raschke M, Riefke B, et al. The involvement of pro-inflammatory cytokines in nephrogenic systemic fibrosis. A mechanistic hypothesis based on preclinical results from a rat model treated with gadodiamide. Exp Toxicol Pathol, in press.

63. Edward M, Quinn JA, Mukherjee S, et al. Gadodiamide contrast agent 'activates' fibroblasts: a possible cause of nephrogenic systemic fibrosis. J Pathol 2008;214(5):584–93.

64. Varani J, DaSilva M, Warner RL, et al. Effects of gadolinium-based magnetic resonance imaging contrast agents on human skin in organ culture and human skin fibroblasts. Invest Radiol 2009; 44(2):74–81.

65. Kuo PH. NSF-active and NSF-inert species of gadolinium: mechanistic and clinical implications. Am J Roentgenol 2008;191(6):1861–3.

66. Fazeli A, Lio PA, Liu V. Nephrogenic fibrosing dermopathy: are ACE inhibitors the missing link? Arch Dermatol 2004;140(11):140–1.

67. Wermuth PJ, Del Galdo F, Jiménez SA. Induction of the expression of profibrotic cytokines and growth factors in normal human peripheral blood monocytes by gadolinium contrast agents. Arthritis Rheum 2009;60(5):1508–18.

68. Harpur ES, Worah D, Hals PA, et al. Preclinical safety assessment and pharmacokinetics of gadodiamide injection, a new magnetic resonance imaging contrast agent. Invest Radiol 1993; 28(Suppl 1):S28–43.

69. Wible JH, Troup CM, Hynes MR, et al. Toxicological assessment of gadoversetamide injection (OptiMARK), a new contrast-enhancement agent for use in magnetic resonance imaging. Invest Radiol 2001;36(7):401–12.

70. Günzel P, Müller N. Toxicology of contrast media for magnetic resonance imaging. A brief review. Adv Magn Reson Imaging Contrast 1992;1(Suppl 1): 29–36.

71. Sieber M, Pietsch H, Walter J, et al. A preclinical study to investigate the development of nephrogenic systemic fibrosis: a possible role for gadolinium-based contrast media. Invest Radiol 2008;43(1):65–75.

72. Pietsch H, Lengsfeld P, Steger-Hartmann T, et al. Impact of long-term retention of gadolinium in the rodent skin following the administration of gadolinium-based contrast agents. Invest Radiol 2009; 44(4):226–33.

73. Sieber MA, Lengsfeld P, Frenzel T, et al. Preclinical investigation to compare different gadolinium-based contrast agents regarding their propensity to release gadolinium in vivo and to trigger nephrogenic systemic fibrosis. Eur Radiol 2008;18(10):2164–73.

74. Grant D, Johnsen H, Juelsrud A, et al. Effects of gadolinium contrast agents in naive and nephrectomized rats: relevance to nephrogenic systemic fibrosis. Acta Radiol 2009;50(2):156–69.

75. Cowper SE, Rabach M, Girardi M. Clinical and histological findings in nephrogenic systemic fibrosis. Eur J Radiol 2008;66(2):191–9.

76. Abraham JL, Thakral C. Tissue distribution and kinetics of gadolinium and nephrogenic systemic fibrosis. Eur J Radiol 2008;66(2):200–7.

77. High WA, Ayers RA, Chandler J, et al. Gadolinium is detectable within the tissue of patients with nephrogenic systemic fibrosis. J Am Acad Dermatol 2007; 56(1):21–6.

78. Idée JM, Port M, Medina C, et al. Possible involvement of gadolinium chelates in the pathophysiology of nephrogenic systemic fibrosis: a critical review. Toxicology 2008;248(2-3):77–88.

79. Haylor JL, Dencausse A, Vickers M, et al. Increased skin cellularity following Omniscan in rats with reduced renal function. Eur Radiol 2009;19(Suppl 1):S285 [abstract B-621].

80. Edward M, Jardine AG, Quinn JA, et al. Assessment of the ability of gadolinium-based contrast agents to stimulate fibroblast proliferation: a possible link to nephrogenic systemic fibrosis. Eur Radiol 2009; 19(Suppl 1):S285 [abstract B-625].

81. Pardo A, Selman M. MMP-1: the elder in the family. Int J Biochem Cell Biol 2005;37(2):283–8.

82. Checa M, Ruiz V, Montaño M, et al. MMP-1 polymorphisms and the risk of idiopathic pulmonary fibrosis. Hum Genet 2008;124(5):465–72.

83. Brezis M. Forefronts in nephrology: summary of the newer aspects of renal cell injury. Kidney Int 1992; 42(3):523–39.

84. Shieren G, Tokmak F, Lefringhausen L, et al. C-reactive protein levels and clinical symptoms following gadolinium administration in hemodialysis patients. Am J Kidney Dis 2008;51(6):976–86.

How to Avoid Nephrogenic Systemic Fibrosis: Current Guidelines in Europe and the United States

Henrik S. Thomsen, MD[a,b,*]

KEYWORDS

- Gadolinium-based contrast media
- Nephrogenic systemic fibrosis • Guidelines
- Late adverse reactions • Glomerular filtration rate

In the first half of 2006, the first evidence of a link between gadolinium-based contrast agents (Gd-CAs), in particular gadodiamide, and the development of nephrogenic systemic fibrosis (NSF) became apparent.[1–5] The association between the administration of gadolinium diethylene triamine pentacetic acid salt (Gd-DTPA) and the development of NSF was not made until the second half of 2006. In February 2007, the European Medicines Agency (EMEA) contraindicated the use of gadodiamide in patients who have a glomerular filtration rate (GFR) of less than 30 mL/min, and four months later, a caution for its use in patients who have a GFR between 30 and 60 mL/min was added. At the same time, the EMEA decided to contraindicate the use of gadopentetate dimeglumine in patients who have a GFR of less than 30 mL/min and stated that it should only be used with caution in patients who have a GFR between 30 and 60 mL/min.[6] For the first time in radiologic history, renal function was introduced into the summary of product characteristics, which was new for European radiologists. To fulfill the rules, it became necessary to determine the GFR in all patients before using the above-mentioned agents. In the United States, the US Food and Drug Administration, on May 23, 2007, requested that vendors add warnings about the risk for developing NSF to the full prescribing information on the packaging for all Gb-CAs (gadopentetate dimeglumine, gadodiamide, gadoversetamide, gadoteridol, gadobenate dimeglumine).[7] The new labels highlighted and described the risk for NSF following exposure to a Gd-CA in patients who had acute or chronic severe renal insufficiency (GFR <30 mL/min/1.73 m^2) and patients who had acute renal insufficiency of any severity due to hepato-renal syndrome or in the perioperative liver transplantation period. In such patients, the use of a Gd-CA should be avoided unless the diagnostic information is essential and not available using non–contrast-enhanced MRI. NSF may result in fatal or debilitating systemic fibrosis.

CONSEQUENCES

The consequences of the finding of a link between exposure to some Gd-CAs and the development of NSF have been multiple. Some centers have

a Department of Diagnostic Sciences, Faculty of Health Sciences, University of Copenhagen, Blegdamsvej 3B, DK-Copenhagen N, Denmark
b Department of Diagnostic Radiology 54E2, Copenhagen University Hospital Herlev, Herlev Ringvej 75, DK-2370 Herlev, Denmark
* Department of Diagnostic Radiology 54E2, Copenhagen University Hospital Herlev, Herlev Ringvej 75, DK-2370 Herlev, Denmark.
E-mail address: hentho01@heh.regionh.dk

Radiol Clin N Am 47 (2009) 871–875
doi:10.1016/j.rcl.2009.05.002

completely stopped doing enhanced MRI for patients who have a GFR of less than 60 mL/min and now refer such patients to receive enhanced CT and conventional X-ray examinations such as arteriography. Other centers have set the GFR level at 30 mL/min. Some centers have changed to the use of more stable agents, if they did not use them before, and some continue as though nothing has happened. Almost everywhere, the liberal use of Gd-CAs as they were used in the first half of the current decade has ceased.

Is it ethically correct to deny a patient an enhanced MRI examination and to refer that patient to receive some other imaging procedure, such as contrast-enhanced CT? First, there are several diseases in which the diagnostic efficacy of MRI is superior to CT.[8] It does not seem to be correct to refer a patient to an inferior imaging method. Second, what is the cost of not identifying the presence of a disease for the patient because of the use of inferior imaging techniques? This fact is often overlooked in the debate. Third, ionizing radiation is used in CT but not in MRI. Fourth, contrast-enhanced CT involves a risk for inducing contrast medium nephropathy.[9] In patients who have a GFR between 15 and 40 mL/min, the risk is probably around 5%, but in patients who have a GFR of less than 15 mL/min, it is likely to be higher. There are no studies looking at the prevalence of contrast-induced nephropathy in patients who have a GFR that is less than 15 mL/min, but it is widely acknowledged that such patients are at very high risk for this complication with the use of all types of iodinated contrast agents. However, the risk for developing NSF in this patient group after exposure to a macrocyclic agent is close to zero, and probably around 10% after exposure to a nonionic linear chelate. Although NSF can be a devastating disease, contrast-induced nephropathy is also a serious complication that is associated with increased morbidity and even mortality.[3,9–11] Thus, considering the very low risk for inducing NSF with the use of a macrocyclic Gd-CA and the high diagnostic accuracy of MRI, it is more beneficial for a patient who has advanced renal disease to undergo an enhanced MRI examination using a macrocyclic agent than it is for such a patient to receive an enhanced CT examination, with its associated risk for contrast nephropathy.

EUROPEAN GUIDELINES

In October 2007, the European Society of Urogenital Radiology's (ESUR) Contrast Media Safety Committee released its first guidelines for Gd-CA use.[3] In the spring of 2008, those guidelines were modified according to the new classification of Gd-CAs introduced by the EMEA.[12] At time of this article's writing, the committee statement on NSF includes the following guidelines:[13]

Patients at a high risk are those who have chronic kidney disease (CKD) 4 and 5 (GFR <30 mL/min), including those who require dialysis and those who have reduced renal function who have had or are awaiting liver transplantation. Patients who have a lower risk are those who have CKD 3 (GFR 30–59 mL/min) and children younger than 1 year old, because of their immature renal function. Patients who have normal renal function are not at risk for NSF.

The following contrast agents are considered to be of highest risk for NSF: gadodiamide, gadopentetate dimeglumine, and gadoversetamide. The use of these agents is contraindicated in patients who have CKD 4 and 5 (GFR <30 mL/min), including those who require dialysis and patients who have reduced renal function who have had or are awaiting liver transplantation. They should be used with caution in patients who have CKD 3 (GFR 30–59 mL/min) and children younger than 1 year old. Serum creatinine (eGFR) levels should always be measured before using these three agents.

The intermediate-risk group includes the following agents: gadobenate dimeglumine (Similar diagnostic results can be achieved using lower doses because of its 2%–3% protein binding); gadofosveset trisodium (It is a blood pool agent with affinity to albumin. Diagnostic results can be achieved using 50% lower doses than with extracellular Gd-CA. Its biologic half-life is 12 times longer than for extracellular agents [18 hours compared with $1\frac{1}{2}$ hours, respectively]); and gadoxetate disodium (It is an organ-specific Gd-CA with 10% protein binding and 50% excretion by hepatocytes. Diagnostic results can be achieved using lower doses than with extracellular Gd-CAs). The determination of eGFR levels is not mandatory before using these agents.

The low-risk group includes the following agents: gadobutrol, gadoterate meglumine, and gadoteridol. The measurement of eGFR levels before administration is not mandatory.

If two different Gd-CAs are injected, it will be impossible to determine with certainty which agent triggers the development of NSF, and the situation is described as "confounded." However, the agent that is most likely responsible is the one that has triggered NSF in other, unconfounded situations.

The committee recommends in all patients independent of renal function that the smallest amount of contrast medium necessary for a diagnostic result be used. Patients who have a good clinical indication should never be denied an enhanced MRI examination. Finally, the agent that leaves the smallest amount of gadolinium in the body should always be the one that is used.

These guidelines were subsequently adopted by the European Society of Magnetic Resonance in Medicine and Biology (ESMRMB).[14]

GUIDELINES IN NORTH AMERICA

(1) The American College of Radiologists (ACR) MRI Safety group[15] was the first American group to come up with recommendations for Gd-CA use. In 2007, the group concluded that the development of cases of NSF has been associated with the isolated prior administration of gadodiamide at rates that exceeded those associated with simple market share of the products, and that cases had also been associated with the use of gadopentetate dimeglumine and gadoversetamide. Nevertheless, a potential association might exist for all five of the US Food and Drug Administration–approved Gd-CAs used for MRI, until there are more definitive data to suspect otherwise. The group recommended no special treatment or handling of patients who had stage 1 or 2 chronic kidney disease (defined as the presence of kidney damage with GFR >90 mL/min/1.73 m^2 or GFR 60–89 mL/min/1.73 m^2, respectively). The only exception to this is that patients who have any level of renal disease should not receive gadodiamide for their contrast-enhanced MRI examinations. The group does not recommend prospectively checking patient renal function, eGFR levels, or GFR before accepting a patient for an MRI procedure. Instead, it recommends that all requests for MRI should be prescreened using an additional question inquiring about the presence of a history of "kidney disease or dialysis." If the disease is present and severe or end-stage in nature, the patient will often be aware of this level of kidney disease. Alternatively, the administration of any of the agents with which NSF has been most strongly associated can be avoided. In patients who have acute kidney injury (AKI), it was recommended that administration of any Gd-CA should be refrained from unless a risk–benefit assessment for a particular patient indicates that the benefits of doing so clearly outweigh the potential risks. When a risk–benefit assessment warrants administration of a Gd-CA to a patient who has renal disease from stages 3 to 5 (moderate to end-stage) or AKI, consideration should be given to administering the lowest dose that would provide the diagnostic benefit being sought, with a half dose, if clinically acceptable, being considered the default standard dose for such patients. The study should be monitored during its execution and before contrast administration to ensure that the administration of the Gd-CA is still deemed necessary and indicated at that time. Postponing the examination in patients who have AKI until renal function has recovered should also be considered if clinically feasible. The name of the patient, name and specific brand of the Gd-CA, dose, route, and rate of administration should all be explicitly specified on the order, along with the date and signature of the requesting radiologist.

A history of multiple prior Gd-CA administrations or hepato-renal disease also seems to be associated with an increased incidence of subsequent development of NSF. The possibility that the existence of acidosis or active inflammatory or thrombotic processes can be risk factors has been entertained, but has not been reproducibly established at this point. This information should be taken into account during the risk–benefit assessment of each individual patient. For administration of a Gd-CA to patients on hemodialysis, the patient is to be transported to have the hemodialysis performed immediately upon termination of the MRI examination. An additional hemodialysis session should be considered within 24 hours of this first contrast-enhanced treatment session. Before a decision is made, the risks of initiating hemodialysis must be seriously weighed against those of developing NSF in each particular case.

For administration of a Gd-CA for patients on chronic ambulatory peritoneal dialysis (also known as continuous cycler-assisted peritoneal dialysis or automated peritoneal dialysis), there seems to be strong reason for hesitating to administer these agents. This process of dialysis seems to be ineffective at clearing the gadolinium from the body. Thus, special caution should be exercised when deciding whether a patient who is on peritoneal dialysis should receive a Gd-CA.

Finally, the ACR MRI Safety group stressed that withholding clinically indicated Gd-CA use can also be associated with its own risks, which should be considered in the decision-making process for all patients who have kidney disease.

(2) Later, the ACR committee on contrast media[16] presented their guidelines. To identify patients who are at high risk for NSF, it is recommended that all patients be questioned for a history of renal disease. This could be accomplished by obtaining a history or by using laboratory tests. When a high-risk patient is identified, the committee recommends considering the use of alternative studies, informing such patients about the potential risks of Gd-CA–enhanced MRI studies should such studies be deemed necessary despite the risks,

using the lowest possible dose of a Gd-CA required to obtain the needed clinical information, avoiding double- or triple-dose studies if at all possible, and avoiding the use of those Gd-CAs that have been most frequently associated with NSF.

If a contrast-enhanced, cross-sectional imaging study is required in patients who have end-stage renal disease and who are on chronic dialysis, it would be reasonable to consider administering iodinated contrast media and performing a CT examination rather than an MRI examination when such a substitution is deemed possible. If a contrast-enhanced MRI examination must be performed, it should be performed shortly before dialysis because prompt, postprocedural dialysis may reduce the likelihood that NSF will develop, although this has not been proved definitively to date. It may be difficult for a busy dialysis center to alter dialysis schedules at the request of imaging departments. Therefore, it may be more feasible for the imaging studies to be timed to precede a scheduled dialysis session.

The correct course of action in patients who have CKD 4 or 5 (eGFR <30 mL/min/1.73 m^2) and who are not on chronic dialysis is most problematic because administration of iodinated contrast media for CT could worsen renal function and lead to the need for dialysis, whereas administration of a Gd-CA for MRI could lead to NSF. For patients who have a GFR that is less than 15 mL/min, it is recommended that any contrast media administration is avoided if at all possible. If Gd-CA administration is absolutely essential, judicious use of the lowest possible doses of a selected Gd-CA needed to obtain a diagnostic study is probably safest. There is no proof that any Gd-CA is completely safe in the less than 15 mL/min patient group; however, at the present time, should Gd-CA use be required in such patients, some investigators have suggested avoiding the use of gadodiamide and considering the use of macrocyclic agents.

Assuming that an accurate assessment of renal function can be made and that the patient is stable, patients who have CKD 3 (eGFR 30–59 mL/min/1.73 m^2) can be considered to be at extremely low or no risk for developing NSF (as long as a dose of a Gd-CA of 0.1 mmol/kg or less is used).

Currently, there is no evidence that patients who have CKD 1 or 2 (eGFR 60–119 mL/min/1.73 m^2) are at increased risk for developing NSF. The current consensus is that all Gd-CAs can be administered safely to such patients (as long as a dose of 0.1 mmol/kg or less is used).

Administration of iodinated contrast media for CT is to be avoided in patients in acute renal failure because there may otherwise be recoverable renal function. Gd-CAs should only be administered if absolutely necessary. The lowest dose necessary to achieve a diagnostic study should be administered. Again, current evidence suggests that gadodiamide should be avoided in such patients.

SUMMARY

Overall, there are no major differences between the North American and European guidelines for the avoidance of NSF. Everyone agrees that patients who have reduced and, in particular, severely reduced renal function are at risk for developing NSF and that in such patients the use of nonionic linear Gd-CAs should be avoided. The Europeans are more forthcoming about the use of the stable macrocyclic contrast agents in these patients than the Americans, but on both sides of the Atlantic Ocean, it is agreed that a well-indicated examination should not be denied. Overlooking a disease is also an important factor that should be considered.

REFERENCES

1. Grobner T. Gadolinium—a specific trigger for the development of nephrogenic fibrosing dermopathy and nephrogenic systemic fibrosis? Nephrol Dial Transplant 2006;21:1104–8.
2. Marckmann P, Skov L, Rossen K, et al. Nephrogenic systemic fibrosis: suspected etiological role of gadodiamide used for contrast-enhanced magnetic resonance imaging. J Am Soc Nephrol 2006;17:2359–62.
3. Thomsen HS. Nephrogenic systemic fibrosis: a serious late adverse reaction to gadodiamide. Eur Radiol 2006;16:2619–21.
4. Broome DR, Girguis M, Baron P, et al. Gadodiamide-associated nephrogenic systemic fibrosis: why radiologists should be concerned. AJR Am J Roentgenol 2007;188:586–92.
5. Sadowski E, Bennett LK, Chan MR, et al. Nephrogenic systemic fibrosis: risk factors and incidence estimation. Radiology 2007;43:148–57.
6. EMEA. Public assessment report. Increased risk of nephrogenic fibrosing dermopathy/nephrogenic systemic fibrosis and gadolinium-containing MRI contrast agents. June 26th, 2007. Available at: http://www.esur.org/fileadmin/NSF/Public_Assessment_Report_NSF_Gadolinium_26_June_2007.pdf. Accessed April 9, 2009.
7. Kanal E, Broome DR, Martin DR, et al. Response to the FDA's May 23, 2007, nephrogenic systemic fibrosis update. Radiology 2008;246:11–4.

8. Dawson P, Punwani S. Nephrogenic systemic fibrosis: non-gadolinium options for the imaging of CKD/ESRD patients. Semin Dial 2008;21: 160–5.

9. Thomsen HS, Morcos SK, Barrett BJ. Contrast-induced nephropathy: The wheel has turned 360 degrees. Acta Radiol 2008;49:646–57.

10. Thomsen HS. Delayed reactions: nephrogenic systemic fibrosis. In: Thomsen HS, Webb JAW, editors. Contrast media: safety issues and ESUR guidelines. 2nd revised edition. Heidelberg (Germany): Springer Verlag; 2009. p. 187–96.

11. Thomsen HS. Contrast medium–induced nephropathy. In: Thomsen HS, Webb JAW, editors. Contrast media: safety issues and ESUR guidelines. 2nd revised edition. Heidelberg (Germany): Springer Verlag; 2009. p. 63–80.

12. Stenver DI. Pharmacovigilance: what to do if you see an adverse reaction and the consequences. Eur J Radiol 2008;66:184–6.

13. Thomsen HS. Guidelines on contrast media. In: Thomsen HS, Webb JAW, editors. Contrast media: safety issues and ESUR guidelines. 2nd revised edition. Heidelberg (Germany): Springer Verlag; 2009. p. 229–42.

14. European Society of Magnetic Resonance in Medicine and Biology. ESMRMB recommendations on adverse reactions to gadolinium based on contrast agents. Available at: http://www.esmrmb.org/html/img/pool/ESMRMB__recommendation_on_NSF.pdf. Accessed April 9, 2009.

15. Kanal E, Barkovich AJ, Bell C, et al. ACR blue ribbon panel on MR safety. ACR guidance document for safe MR practices: 2007. AJR Am J Roentgenol 2007;188:1447–74.

16. American College of Radiology. Manual on contrast media version 6.0 with changes until September 2008. Available at: http://www.acr.org/SecondaryMainMenuCategories/quality_safety/contrast_manual.aspx. Accessed April 9, 2009.

Index

Note: Page numbers of article titles are in **boldface** type.

Radiol Clin N Am 47 (2009) 877–878
doi:10.1016/S0033-8389(09)00141-9
0033-8389/09/$ – see front matter © 2009 Elsevier Inc. All rights reserved.

radiologic.theclinics.com

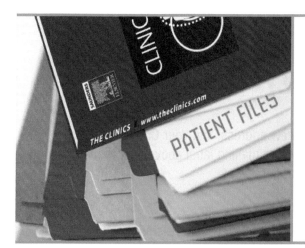
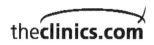

Moving?

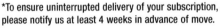

Make sure your subscription moves with you!

To notify us of your new address, find your **Clinics Account Number** (located on your mailing label above your name), and contact customer service at:

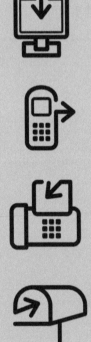

Email: journalscustomerservice-usa@elsevier.com

800-654-2452 (subscribers in the U.S. & Canada)
314-447-8871 (subscribers outside of the U.S. & Canada)

Fax number: 314-447-8029

Elsevier Health Sciences Division
Subscription Customer Service
3251 Riverport Lane
Maryland Heights, MO 63043

*To ensure uninterrupted delivery of your subscription,
please notify us at least 4 weeks in advance of move.

Printed and bound by CPI Group (UK) Ltd, Croydon, CR0 4YY

03/10/2024

01040362-0007